Basic Method Validation

Validation

3rd Edition

James O. Westgard, PhD

with contributions from

Patricia L. Barry, BS, MT(ASCP)
R. Neill Carey, PhD, FACB
Sharon S. Ehrmeyer, PhD
Elsa F. Quam, BS, MT(ASCP)
Sten Westgard, MS

Copyright © 2008

Westgard QC, Inc.
7614 Gray Fox Trail
Madison WI 53717
Phone 608-833-4718 Fax 608-833-0640
http://www.westgard.com

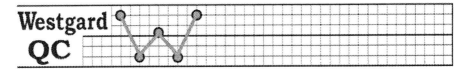

Library of Congress Control Number: 2008927458
ISBN 1-886958-25-4
ISBN13: 9781886958258
Published by Westgard QC, Inc.
7614 Gray Fox Trail
Madison, WI 53717

Phone 608-833-4718

Foreword to the 3rd edition

Basic Method Validation is part of a trilogy of "back to basics" books that focus on analytical quality management. The other two books are *Basic QC Practices* and *Basic Planning for Quality*. When I teach these materials, I start with method validation because it introduces the basic concepts of analytical performance and the experimental and statistical techniques needed to describe performance in quantitative terms. These concepts carry through into the practice of QC and the selection of optimal QC procedures via quality design and planning.

The original source of this approach to method validation goes back thirty years to a series of papers that were published in the *American Journal of Medical Technology* and later as a monograph titled *Method Evaluation*. My co-authors were Diane J de Vos, Marian R. Hunt, Else F. Quam, R. Neill Carey, and Carl C. Garber, all of whom worked at the University of Wisconsin. We introduced this approach at workshops that were taught at the national ASMT and AACC meetings. Today Neill and Carl, together with David Koch, continue to teach this approach at the AACC national meeting. They now hold the record for the longest running workshop in AACC history.

This 3rd edition provides important updates based on new regulatory requirements and emerging standards of practice, particularly the latest guidelines from CLSI (Clinical and Laboratory Standards Institute):

- Updated CLIA regulations and accreditation requirements;

- Revised chapter on reportable range that includes calibration verification;

- Revised chapter on detection limits that includes concepts of Limit of Blank, Limit of Detection, and Limit of Quantitation, as recommended in the CLSI EP17 guideline;

- Updated "Method Decision Chart" that includes criteria for 2, 3, 4, 5, and 6-Sigma performance;

- New chapter on estimation of trueness and precision based on the CLSI EP15-A2 guideline, including directions for performing the required calculations using electronic spreadsheets;

- New chapter on evolving global standards (ISO, International Standards Organization), ISO 15189, and the concepts of trueness and measurement uncertainty.

- New chapter on Six Sigma metrics, including instructions on how to convert method validation data into Sigma metrics.

For more than thirty years, I have worked on quality control and method validation. While statistics, equations and calculations may not change, the context and the environment are constantly evolving. I hope this third edition helps you understand these method validation numbers in the proper context of your laboratory.

James O. Westgard
Madison Wisconsin

Acknowledgments

First and foremost, Sten Westgard deserves the credit for the "formula" used in developing these materials. He is responsible for the publication of these materials and also provides a driving force for their completion. At my age, I need deadlines to get things finished and I get them from Sten.

Several colleagues have helped in the development of these materials, including Elsa Quam and Patricia Barry who are long-time associates of mine in the Clinical Laboratories at the University of Wisconsin Hospital and Clinics. Sharon Ehrmeyer continues to help clarify the wonderful world of CLIA rules, regulations, and related accreditation and inspection guidelines. Neill Carey contributed his experience and knowledge to make the presentation of the EP15 guidelines practical and useful.

The antique maps that appear in this book are part of a small personal collection. I hope you find them helpful for illustrating key ideas in the book, as well as interesting and beautiful historical documents.

About the authors and contributors

James O. Westgard, PhD, FACB is an Emeritus Professor in the Department of Pathology and Laboratory Medicine at the University of Wisconsin Medical School, where he continues to teach in the Clinical Laboratory Science program.

Patricia L. Barry, BS, MT(ASCP), is a Quality Specialist in the Clinical Laboratories at the University of Wisconsin Hospital and Clinics.

R. Neill Carey, PhD, FACB is Director of Special Chemistry at Peninsula Regional Medical Center, Salisbury, Maryland.

Sharon S. Ehrmeyer, PhD, MT(ASCP), is a Professor in the Department of Pathology and Laboratory Medicine and Director of the Clinical Laboratory Science Program at the University of Wisconsin Medical School.

Elsa F. Quam, BS, MT(ASCP), is a Quality Specialist in the Clinical Laboratories at the University of Wisconsin Hospital and Clinics.

Sten Westgard, BA, MS, is the Director of Client Services and Technology for Westgard QC, Inc.

There's more online at Westgard Web

In order to squeeze in all the updates, revisions, and entirely new chapters into this book, yet still keep it a reasonable length, we had to make some cuts. Notably, we had to cut out the glossary and reference lists

But don't worry, you can still view these resources if you need them.

Go to **http://www.westgard.com/bmv/extras.html** for access and links to these features:

- Frequently-Asked-Questions (FAQs)

- Glossary of terms

- Complete reference list for this book

- Links to spreadsheets, worksheets and other downloads

- Links to Method Validation calculators, including some calculators not available to the general public.

Table of Contents

1. **Is quality still an issue for laboratory tests?** 1
   - Myths of quality 3
2. **How do you manage quality?** 13
   - The need for standard processes and standards of quality 15
3. **What is the purpose of a method validation study?** 27
   - MV – The inner, hidden, deeper, secret meaning 28
4. **What are the regulatory requirements for basic method validation?** 37
   - MV – The regulations, by Sharon S. Ehrmeyer, PhD 38
5. **How is a method selected?** 51
   - MV – Selecting a method to validate 52
6. **What experiments are necessary to validate method performance?** 61
   - MV – The experimental plan 62
7. **How are the experimental data analyzed?** 71
   - MV – The data analysis tool kit 72
8. **How are the statistics calculated?** 83
   - MV – The statistical calculations 84
9. **How is the reportable range of a method determined?** 101
   - MV – The linearity or reportable range experiment 102
   - Problem set – Cholesterol method validation data 112
10. **How is the imprecision of a method determined?** 113
    - MV – The replication experiment 114
    - Problem set – Cholesterol method validation data 122
11. **How is the inaccuracy (bias) of a method determined?** ... 123
    - MV – The comparison of method experiments 124
    - Problem set – Cholesterol method validation data 135
12. **How do you use statistics to estimate analytical errors?** 137
    - MV – Statistical sense, sensitivity, and significance 138
13. **How do you test for specific sources of inaccuracy?** 153
    - MV – The interference and recovery experiments 154
    - Problem set – Cholesterol method validation data 165

14. **What is the lowest test value that is reliable?** **167**
    MV – The detection limit experiment 168
    Problem set – Cholesterol method validation data 175

15. **How is a reference interval verified?** **177**
    MV – Reference interval transference 178

16. **How do you judge the performance of a method?** **187**
    MV – The decision on method performance 188

17. **What's a practical procedure for validating a method?** ... **197**
    MV – The real world applications 198
    MV – The worksheets 207

18. **How do you use statistics in the real world?** **211**
    Points of care in using statistics for method validation 212

19. **How can a manufacturer's claims be verified?** **221**
    Verifying a claims for precision and trueness 222

20. **How can claims be evaluated on the Sigma-scale?** **241**
    Translating performance claims into Sigma metrics 242

21. **What impact will ISO have on analytical quality?** **251**
    Quality concepts: is it better to be uncertain or in error? 252

22. **Self-Assessment Answers** **273**
    Cholesterol Problem Set answers 300

Appendix 1: CLIA'88 Analytical Quality Requirements **307**

Index **311**

1: Is quality still an issue for laboratory tests?

In this introductory chapter, Dr. Westgard challenges current thinking that analytical quality is better than needed for medical care. Using historical maps that were regarded as the most authoritative and accurate records of the times, he illustrates that popular "truths" can be well documented and widely believed, yet entirely wrong. He sets out the need to define requirements for quality in order to manage quality in a quantitative manner.

Objectives:

○ Begin thinking about quality in a critical way.

○ Recognize that current beliefs about quality may not be grounded in fact.

○ Identify the critical issue for managing quality in a quantitive way.

Lesson materials:

○ **Myths of quality**, by James O. Westgard, PhD

Things to do:

○ Study the lesson.

○ Find out what quality is needed for a cholesterol test.

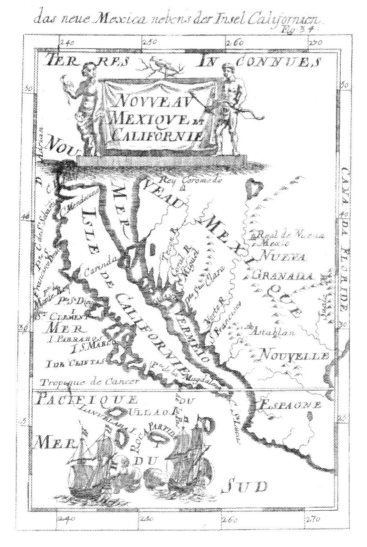

The Mythical Island of California!
NOUVEAU MEXIQUE ET CALIFORNIA, *by Alain Mallet,*
Paris 1686. A miniature French map showing California as a
flat-topped island – a myth that persisted from 1620 for over 100
years.

Myths of Quality

James O. Westgard, PhD

A MYTH is a Mistaken Yarn, Theory, or Hypothesis!

Historical Myths of Cartography

Mythical island of California. Did you know that California was an island? It's well documented on the most reputable maps of the 1600s that California was completely surrounded by water. For example, see the accompanying map that shows the *Isle de Californie*. There it is, documented in black and white, proof that California was an island.

This map of *Nouveau Mexique et Californie* by Alain Mallet was published in 1686 in the *Description de l'Univers* (Paris). Mallet copied the flat-topped model of California that appeared in an earlier map by Sanson, who was one of the most distinguished French cartographers (It was very common for mapmakers to copy each other's work). When a new discovery appeared on one map, it was widely "disseminated" on the other maps of the time. The discovery that California was an island was first documented in 1622 and persisted on maps as late as 1750, even though evidence in 1705 clearly established that this was a myth.

Mythical island of Friesland. Actually, there is quite a history of mythical islands, suggesting that these myths are not as rare as you might expect. In the late 1500s, one of the most famous mapmakers, Abraham Ortelius, prepared a map of the Northern Atlantic that showed an island of Friesland lying a bit west and south of Iceland, complete with a detailed description of the coastline, the harbors, the people who lived there, what they looked like, and what they did for a living. It's a beautiful map, decorated with sailing ships and sea creatures, and was the most authoritative map of the area at that time. The only problem was that Friesland didn't exist. When people sailed to the new world and passed Iceland, they ascribed more and more details and reality to Friesland because they expected it was the next body of land.

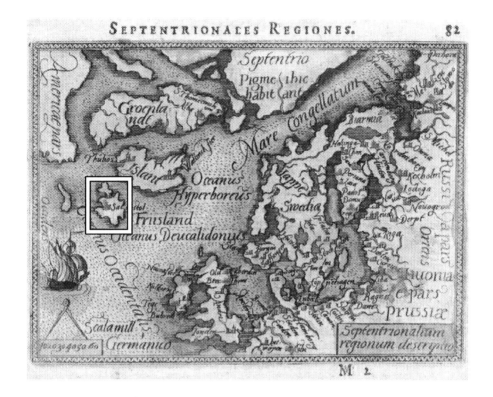

The mythical island of Friesland!
SEPTENTRIONALES REGIONES, *by Philip Galle, Antwerp, 1595. A miniature of Ortelius' famous map of the north Atlantic region showing the mythical island of Friesland (see box) located to the southwest of Iceland.*

Mythical islands in Lake Superior. Another example that is of interest to those of us in the midwest are the islands of Ponchartrain and Phillipeaux in Lake Superior. When the border between the U.S. and Canada was settled by the Treaty of Paris in 1783, it was decided that these islands would be part of the U.S. In the early 1800s when Wisconsin was being settled, the U.S. government sent out surveyors to map this area more completely, but they couldn't find these islands! They appeared on all the maps of the time, but they didn't show up above the water. It seems that the explorers created these islands and named them for the government minister who was funding their investigations. They were probably trying to get more funding for further explorations and needed some preliminary findings to justify more money.

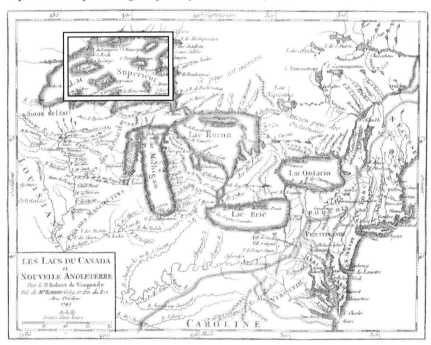

The mythical islands in Lake Superior!
LES LACS DU CANADA et NOUVELLE ANGLETERRE, *by Robert de Vaugondy, Paris, 1749. This map shows Lac Superieur containing the real Isle Royale and the mythical islands of Phillipeaux, Pontchartrain, Maurepas, St. Anne.*

Modern myths of quality

These cartographic myths are amusing in retrospect, but they were taken very seriously at the time and created problems later on. There are myths today that are also taken seriously and will cause us serious problems in the future. Some of them hit very close to home – the quality of healthcare and the quality of laboratory testing.

Myth: QA assures quality in healthcare. It's a *mistaken yarn* that puts a good spin on current efforts to measure the quality of healthcare. As healthcare providers, we all talk about quality assurance (QA), but our quality assurance programs (which are often required by regulation and accreditation) primarily deal with measuring performance. Quality Assessment would be a better name for these efforts. While it is important to **assess** quality to know how well we're doing, measuring quality doesn't **assure** that the necessary quality will be achieved. Achieving quality actually requires quality design and planning, which starts with defining the quality that is needed, then builds that quality into the process.

Myth: Statistical QC controls the quality of laboratory tests. It's a *mistaken theory* that the use of statistics somehow assures that laboratory test results have the necessary quality. Virtually all laboratories apply statistical quality control (QC) as part of their efforts to assure the quality of laboratory tests. While we may not understand the theory or the statistics, we still believe that something magical happens because of those statistics. Somehow by analyzing controls and plotting results on control charts, we expect to control the quality of our testing processes, even if we don't understand how it works.

Myth: Quality can be managed even if the required quality isn't known. It's a *mistaken hypothesis* that quality can be managed when we don't know the quality that is needed. Few laboratories have defined the analytical quality that is needed for the tests they perform. How is it possible to know we are achieving the unknown? Can you manage the finances of the laboratory without knowing the budget? Don't you need to know the quality required for a laboratory test if you are to manage the quality of the testing process?

Myth: Quality requirements need to consider only impre-cision and inaccuracy. This problem with quality requirements gets to be even more complicated. Current thinking about quality goals and requirements is flawed because it considers only the stable method performance characteristics (imprecision and inaccuracy). If perfor-mance is stable, why bother doing quality control at all? If QC is necessary, don't we have to consider the performance characteristics of QC procedures (probabilities for error detection and false rejection) in our goal setting models?

Myth: Current laboratory methods have better impreci-sion and inaccuracy than needed. The net effect of all these myths is the belief that the performance of current laboratory methods is better than required for medical needs. This belief is based on a mistaken theory for setting quality goals, a mistaken hypothesis in equating all medically tolerable variation with ana-lytical variation, disregarding the subject's own biological varia-tion, and the mistaken assumption that QC procedures have ideal response curves and can detect any change in performance, regard-less how small.

Myth: Analytical quality is a given today. As a conse-quence of these myths, there is a common feeling today that analytical quality is a given, i.e., analytical quality itself is being assumed today. In the midst of programs on Six Sigma, Lean, Risk Management, and Total Quality Management (TQM), it is often mistakenly assumed that the problems in technical quality manage-ment have already been solved. This represents the mistaken hypoth-esis that past efforts have resolved any technical difficulties, so now we can get on to new issues that are in vogue, such as monitoring customer satisfaction, measuring patient outcomes, etc.

Myth: No further improvements in analytical quality are needed. The collective result of all these myths is a false sense of security regarding the quality of laboratory testing processes. Many think analytical quality is so good that there is no need for further improvements. This is the most serious myth of all because it makes us complacent about what we are doing and hinders efforts to further improve the analytical quality of laboratory tests.

Myth: The government regulates laboratory tests to make sure quality is acceptable. While it is true that the Food and Drug Administration (FDA) does approve new tests and analytic systems, it is important to understand that this clearance is based only on "truth in labeling." Manufacturers are required to make claims for certain performance characteristics, such as reportable range, precision, accuracy, interference, detection limit, and reference range and to submit data to support those claims. The FDA's process focuses on whether or not the data supports the manufacturers' claims, not whether or not the quality of the testing process is acceptable for patient care. We may believe that manufacturers would not submit a new test for FDA clearance unless the quality was acceptable, but that assumption is not always true.

Myth: Laboratories today should focus and pre-analytic and post-analytic errors since analytic errors are no longer a problem. This idea surfaced in 1990 from the CDC in an effort to broaden the quality assessment efforts in clinical laboratories. Later in the 90s, CMS adopted that perspective in revising the CLIA Final Rules to include quality management of the "total testing process," i.e., pre-analytic, analytic, and post-analytic parts of the testing methodology. By the early years of the 21st century, this belief was widely held in the laboratory community and today is used (and accepted) as an argument for reducing the amount of statistical QC performed during the analytic phase. It satisfies our yearning to do less QC, to simplify laboratory testing, and to reduce costs and eliminate trouble-shooting and repeat analyses, all of which allow laboratory tests to be performed in testing sites where technical skills and laboratory experience may be lacking.

Where's the evidence?

In this age of Evidence-Based Laboratory Medicine, where's the data to support these beliefs that we no longer need to worry about analytical quality? While it would take lots of pages in this book to disprove this whole set of mistaken beliefs, let's consider this last myth – laboratories should focus and pre-analytic and post-analytic phases of the total testing process – because it rests on many of the other beliefs. In fact, it would be the logical outcome if analytical errors were truly no longer a problem.

First, let's consider a more complete model for the total testing process, as provided by Goldschmidt et al[1] and shown in the accompanying figure. Called a "filter model," the figure illustrates a series of filters through which a laboratory test request, specimen, and sample must pass. In reality, these are mathematical filters, rather than paper filters as suggested in the figure, but as laboratory scientists rather than mathematicians, the approach is easy to understand from the illustration. This more detailed model describes 5 phases or filters for validating the total testing process.

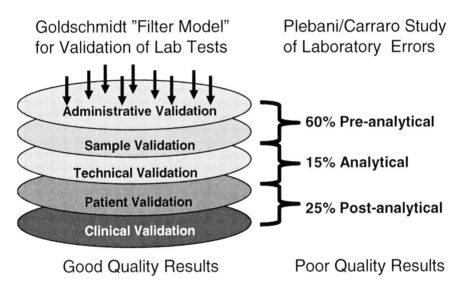

- Administrative validation refers to steps beginning with the selection and ordering of the right test, collection of the right information to understand the context of the test, as well as validation of right patient conditions, right preparation, etc.

- Sample validation is concerned with obtaining the right specimen at the right time on the right patient, the right processing and transportation of the sample, and the right use of that sample for analytical measurements;

- Technical validation has to do with getting the right answer, which requires knowing the quality required for a test, validating the precision and accuracy of measurement process, designing the right QC procedure, and implementing the measurement and control procedures properly;

- Patient validation requires that right test result be correctly reported to the right patient record and considers whether that test result is consistent with knowledge about the patient, other test results on that patient, within the expected variation of the individual patient and the appropriate population group, as well as relationship to critical or alert values, and consistency with patient populations;

- Clinical validation is concerned with the patient receiving the right clinical treatment based on the laboratory test results and services. Clinical validation goes beyond what is normally considered to be part of the validation of test results in the US.

This is a European model and demonstrates that patient and clinical validation have long been a critical part of the validation of laboratory tests. Patient and clinical validation are important professional responsibilities of MD and PhD level laboratory physicians and scientists. With increasing workload, they have developed computerized tools and programs to standardize and facilitate this "medical review" or "medical QC." The importance of the first step (administrative validation) becomes clear in the context of the information needed to complete this medical review and control.

Next, let's consider the most recent and definitive study on the sources of laboratory errors [2]. Drs. Plebani and Carraro have studied laboratory errors for many years and are recognized as leaders in performing such studies. Their results document the distribution of errors shown in figure. Clearly there are more pre-analytic errors (60%) than post-analytic errors (25%) than analytic errors (15%). Many clinical laboratory scientists cite these figures to support the idea that pre-analytic and post-analytic errors are more important than analytic errors and often conclude that analytic quality is no longer an issue.

However, a more detailed reading of the study shows that from the total of 51,746 tests, there were 393 questionable results, 160 of which were confirmed as laboratory errors. Of these 160 errors, 46 caused inappropriate patient care, and 24 of those cases of inappropriate patient care were caused by analytical errors. That means that over half the cases (52%) of inappropriate patient care are due to analytical errors. Analytical errors are still the largest and most important source of errors that cause harm to patients!

We need to recognize that the core competency of a laboratory must be to get the correct test result. All sources of error in the testing process must be carefully managed and monitored, but it must start with analytical errors. If we can't, don't, or won't assure analytical quality of our test results, then we should not be in the business of providing laboratory testing services.

What's the point?

You need to think critically about quality and recognize that many of our current beliefs are not grounded in fact, i.e., not based on scientific evidence. These myths need to be exposed if the technical management of analytical testing processes is to be improved.

That's the purpose of this introduction! You need to critically assess many of the quality management practices that are accepted in laboratories today. To begin, you need to understand how quality requirements can be defined, how method performance should be measured experimentally, how the experimental data can be analyzed with statistics to estimate analytical performance characteristics, and how a decision on the acceptability can be made.

Once the performance of a method has been judged to be acceptable (Basic Method Validation), you need to select a statistical QC procedure that can detect medically important errors (Quality Planning or Quality Design), make routine measurements on the necessary number of controls, and interpret the control results using the appropriate decision criteria or control rules (Basic QC Practices).

References

1. Oosterhuis WP, Ulenkate HJLM, Goldschmidt HMJ. Evaluation of LabRespond, a new automated validation system for clinical laboratory test results. Clin Chem 2001;46:1811-1817.

2. Carraro P, Plebani M. Errors in a Stat Laboratory: Types and frequencies 10 years later. Clin Chem 2007;53:1338 - 1342.

Self-Assessment Questions:

○ What myths of quality exist in laboratories today?

○ What can be done to improve laboratory quality management practices?

2: How do you manage quality?

The principles of Total Quality Management (TQM) are adapted to define a framework for managing quality in a healthcare laboratory. This framework identifies five major components that are needed in a quality management process to provide continuous improvement of quality.

Objectives:

- ○ Identify the major components for managing quality.
- ○ Explain the purpose of each component.
- ○ Give examples of activities associated with each component.
- ○ Recognize the central driving force in this quality management process.
- ○ Describe the role of method validation in this quality management process.

Lesson materials:

- ○ **Management of quality – The need for standard processes and standards of quality**, by James O. Westgard, PhD

Things to do:

- ○ Study the lesson.

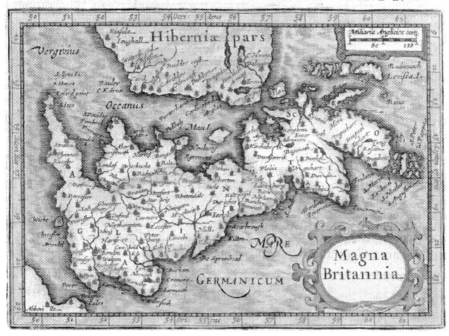

A different perspective!
MAGNA BRITANNIA, *by Petrus Bertius, London 1616.*

This map of England is oriented with North to the right, which provides a different perspective or different view from what we are accustomed to today. You probably found it difficult and confusing to initially recognize the shape of England because we're used to seeing it turned 90 degrees. At the time when this map was published, there was no "standard" orientation that required North to be at the top. The need for standards is what this chapter is about.

Management of Quality:
The Need for Standard Processes and Standards of Quality

James O. Westgard, PhD

Quality must be assured, not assumed! As illustrated in the previous chapter, ideas about the current state of quality in healthcare and laboratory testing may be influenced by **m**istaken **y**arns, theories, and **h**ypotheses, i.e., **myths** that are not supported by fact or data. Quality doesn't just happen! Quality must be achieved by work processes that are carefully planned, properly operated, optimally controlled, appropriately measured, and continuously improved, i.e., by proper management of quality. This lesson emphasizes the need for standard laboratory processes to provide consistent quality, as well as standards of quality to guide the management of those processes.

Standard, standard process, standard of quality

Standard has many meanings in the laboratory. In analytical terms, a *standard solution* provides a known value for calibration of a testing process and represents purity, truth, and correctness. In management terms, a *standard process* provides a consistent way of doing things, e.g., a *standard testing process* provides a well-defined protocol for performing a laboratory test. Likewise, a *standard method validation process* provides a regular and systematic way for evaluating the performance of a laboratory testing process. [Note that the idea of "process" can be applied to any repeated activity, whether physical or mental; both physical work processes and management decision processes need to be standardized or systematized to assure consistent and reliable results.]

Another important term is *standard of quality* which is a criterion or statement that describes the acceptable level of some characteristic. For an analytical test, we need to know how quickly a test result needs to be reported, as well as how close the result must be to the true or correct value. A standard for turnaround time is more easily understood than a standard for truth or correctness.

Page 15

For example, it is obvious that turnaround time should be stated in units of time, usually minutes. These units are understood by both the party requesting the test and the party providing the service. The party ordering the test defines the requirement on the basis of the medical service being provided. Both parties can measure whether the observed performance satisfies the requirement.

Analytical quality is more difficult because it involves technical concepts such as imprecision and inaccuracy, which are not always understood by laboratorians and are certainly less understood by the physicians who order the tests or the patients who are the ultimate consumers of the test results. Customers and consumers of laboratory services cannot easily define the analytical quality that is required (at least not in the analytical terms desired by the laboratory), nor can they measure or assess analytical quality. The laboratory, therefore, must take full responsibility for managing the analytical quality of its services

A standard process for managing quality

Quality management should be a standard laboratory process. Such a process can be structured as shown in the accompanying figure [1]. Beginning at the top and proceeding clockwise, QP refers to quality planning, QLP stands for quality laboratory processes, QC stands for quality control, QA for quality assessment, and QI for quality improvement. In the center, QS stands for quality standards, i.e., standards for the quality required by the test or service being provided.

This framework provides a quality management process that functions like a feedback loop. QP plans the best way to get the work done, e.g., the selection and evaluation of the analytical methods, equipment, reagents, and procedures used to perform laboratory tests;

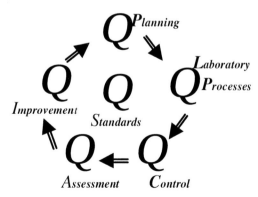

QLP establishes standard work processes to utilize the policies, procedures, protocols, and personnel of the laboratory; QC provides quantitative measures of process performance using statistical process control techniques; QA provides broader measures of how well the work is getting done, e.g., effectiveness of specimen acquisition procedures, turnaround time for laboratory services, appropriate formats for reporting results, etc. When problems are detected, QI provides a problem-solving mechanism to determine root causes, which can then be eliminated through QP, in that case actually re-planning the testing processes and implementing new and better ways of doing the work (i.e., changes in QLP). Through this framework, continuous improvement is built into the management process by cycling through the Q's. Customer focus is achieved by centering these Q's on "quality standards" that represent the laboratory's goals, objectives, and customer requirements – essential information for the objective and quantitative management of the laboratory.

The initial focus of the laboratory is on the establishment of standard operating procedures or processes by which the work gets done. In particular, we are concerned with the selection, validation, and implementation of analytical methods that will provide consistently reliable analytical quality. Those activities are part of QP and lead to the establishment of quality testing processes that are part of QLP. QC is applied after appropriate testing processes have been established. Likewise, QA and QI are part of the ongoing monitoring and improvement of standard operating processes.

Priorities in developing a standard quality management process

Traditional practices for laboratory quality management have always started with establishing standard methods for performing laboratory tests (QLP), then emphasized statistical quality control to monitor analytical performance (QC), and later expanded and broadened the measures of quality to include turnaround time, etc. (QA). Practices of quality improvement (QI) have been introduced as part of Total Quality Management (TQM) or Continuous Quality Improvement (CQI) [2,3] as well as Six Sigma [15].

What is usually lacking in laboratories are:

- Quality Standards (QS): defined quality goals, objectives, and customer requirements, and

- Quality Planning (QP): methodology and skills to build the desired quality into the laboratory processes.

If these quality requirements and the plans for achieving them have not been spelled out, then quality isn't really being managed. Instead, what happens is what happens. It's like the cartoon where Lucky Eddy and Hagar the Horrible are standing at the bar. Hagar asks Lucky Eddy what he'll have, and Lucky Eddy replies "My usual." Hagar asks "What's your usual?" and Lucky Eddy answers "It's what I usually have." In healthcare laboratories, in spite of supposedly well-established management practices of QLP, QC, QA, and TQM, what happens with quality is usually what has happened before. To actually manage quality, laboratories must define the quality that is required and implement systematic processes to validate method performance, select appropriate statistical QC procedures, and monitor process performance in quantitative and objective ways.

A Short History of Quality Standards

Actually, there is a long history of discussion of quality standards in the clinical chemistry literature. Beginning in 1963, a Canadian clinical chemist by the name of David Tonks suggested that the errors that are allowable in a test should be related to the width of the reference interval (at that time called "normal range")[4]. A test having a narrow reference interval should also have high precision in order to distinguish whether a patient was "normal" or not. Tonks recommended that the allowable error for a test should be no larger than a quarter of the normal range.

In 1968, Dr. Roy Barnett, a clinical pathologist, investigated the relationship between the precision performance of laboratory methods and the medical use and interpretation of test results by physicians. In his landmark paper on the "Medical Significance of Laboratory Results" [5], Barnett provided specific guidelines for medically allowable standard deviations (SD) for many common laboratory tests.

Because Tonks defined desirable quality in the form of an allowable error, whereas Barnett defined it in the form of an allowable standard deviation, there was disagreement about the correct way to format recommendations for quality standards. In 1976, the College of American Pathologists convened a conference to discuss analytical goals. As a young clinical chemist who had written papers on method evaluation and the need for quality standards to judge acceptability of new methods, I was invited to present at this conference. I proposed a "total error" concept and the use of "allowable total error" as the best format for defining quality, but found myself on the opposite side of the thinking of well-established clinical chemists and pathologists. The proceedings of this "Aspen Conference" provide some glimpses of the arguments and disagreements [6]. They went on for many years and inhibited the practical application of any form of quality standard in clinical laboratories. During this time, the concept of total error took hold and became accepted in clinical laboratories. Finally in 1999, the Stockholm Consensus Conference brought together many experts in the field to "set global analytical quality specifications" [7]. The outcome was a recommendation for a hierarchy of "quality specifications" to prioritize the preferred source of information, as follows:

- "Evaluation of the effect of analytical performance on clinical outcomes in specific clinical settings;

- Evaluation of the effect of analytical performance on clinical decisions in general:

  - Data based on components of biological variation;

  - Data based on the analysis of clinicians opinions;

- Published professional recommendations:

  - From national and international expert groups;

  - From expert local groups or individuals;

- Performance goals set by

    - Regulatory bodies;

    - Organizers of External Quality Assessment (EQA) schemes;

- Goals based on the current state of the art:

    - As demonstrated by data from EQA or Proficiency Testing schemes;

    - As found in current publications on methodology."

"When available, and when appropriate for the intended purpose, models higher in the hierarchy are to be preferred to those at lower levels." [7] Therefore, specific clinical models are preferred to general clinical models, which in turn are preferred over recommendations from expert groups, criteria from Proficiency Testing or External Quality Assessment programs, and "state of the art" guidelines. In practice, however, a laboratory may have to satisfy regulatory requirements, which then take priority over the clinical models and biologic goals, even though PT and EQC criteria rank lower in the hierarchy.

One final note: terminology varies widely, over time, between scientists, from one text to another, between professions, between parties involved in regulating quality, between countries, between continents, worldwide. You must adapt to different names and terms as you read, study, and search the literature for guidance. I tend to use the terms "quality goals" and "quality requirements" as synonyms for "standards of quality" and reserve the term *specifications* for the precision and accuracy needed to achieve the goal, as in "operating specifications." But much of my earlier writings will show the use of "quality standards," as reflected in this book. Sorry for the confusion, but it is an integral part of the history of quality standards!

Getting started with quality standards

Our objective here is not to have you become an expert in quality standards, but to help you start learning about quality standards and make sure you are aware of different sources of information that are conveniently available. There is no "one and only" way to define the quality needed for a laboratory test, even though there are fierce arguments for and against certain types of quality requirements. Different types of quality standards are needed to manage quality at different places in the process, such as clinical outcome criteria that reflect medically important changes in test results, analytical outcome criteria that describe the allowable total analytical error in test results, and analytical operating specifications that describe the allowable imprecision, allowable bias, and the QC needed to detect medically important errors in the testing process.

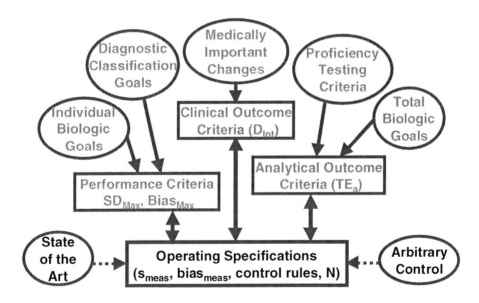

The accompanying figure shows the relationships between certain kinds of recommendations and different types of quality criteria. Starting at the top of the figure, medically important changes in test results can be defined by standard treatment guidelines (clinical pathways, clinical practice guidelines, etc.) to establish clinical outcome criteria (or decision intervals, D_{int}). Such clinical criteria can be converted to laboratory operating specifications for imprecision (s_{meas}), inaccuracy ($bias_{meas}$), and QC (control rules, N) by a clinical quality-planning model [8] that takes into account pre-analytical factors, such as individual or within-subject biologic variation (s_{wsub}).

The right side of the figure shows how proficiency testing criteria define analytical outcome criteria in the form of allowable total errors (TE_a), which can likewise be translated into operating specifications (s_{meas}, $bias_{meas}$, control rules, N) via an analytical quality-planning model [9]. Note that the allowable total error can also be set on the basis of total biologic goals that are population-based or individual-based, therefore the extensive database of individual biologic variation can also be used in this situation [10].

The left side of the figure shows how performance criteria for imprecision and inaccuracy can be defined as separate analytical goals for the maximum imprecision and bias that would be allowable for the stable performance of the method. Specifications for maximum imprecision can be derived on the basis of within-subject biological variation [11]. The maximum allowable bias can be derived from diagnostic classification models [12]. Laboratories can utilize these individual performance criteria by relating observed method performance to the maximum allowable value, calculating the critical-size error that needs to be detected to maintain satisfactory performance, and then selecting appropriate QC procedures by use of power function graphs [10].

The bottom of the figure shows what happens in the absence of any defined standards of quality. "State of the art" analytical performance sets the specifications for imprecision and inaccuracy because manufacturers set their product performance goals on the basis of the performance needed to be competitive in the marketplace. Arbitrary control exists instead of quality control because QC practices are set on the basis of professional practice, regulatory, or accreditation guidelines.

Convenient sources of quality standards

❍ A list of analytical quality requirements is provided by the proficiency testing criteria for acceptable performance that have been defined in the Clinical Laboratory Improvement Amendments (CLIA). This information is readily available and can be used when validating the performance of analytical methods.

See Appendix 1 or **http://www.westgard.com/clia.htm**.

❍ Some information on medically important changes in test results is also available, however, that information needs to be carefully interpreted if used for validating the performance of analytical methods.

See **http://www.westgard.com/clinical.htm**

❍ An extensive online database is available that summarizes all available studies on biologic variation and provides recommendations for precision, bias, and total error specifications. This database is an update of the original work published by Dr. Carmen Ricos and her Spanish colleagues [13]. For the definitive discussion of biologic variation, see the book by Dr. Callum Fraser [14].

See **http://www.westgard.com/biodatabase1.htm**

❍ You can also review earlier European recommendations for biologic goals for imprecision and inaccuracy, as well as calculated biologic allowable total errors, based on individual or within-subject biological variation.

See **http://www.westgard.com/europe.htm**

What's the point?

Method validation should be a standard process in your laboratory. It should be part of your standard operating procedures for getting the work done in your laboratory. That means having a protocol that defines a standard set of experimental procedures, standard ways to collect and analyze the data, and a standard way of judging the acceptability of a new method. And that decision on acceptability depends on defining quality standards that provide objective statements of how good a test should be! A practical starting point for quality standards will be any regulatory requirements that define "criteria for acceptable performance," such as the CLIA requirements for proficiency testing. But the number of tests on the CLIA list is limited and other sources and recommendations will need to be considered, such as those based on within-subject and between-subject biologic variability and, when available, requirements based on the intended clinical use of laboratory tests.

These lessons on method validation will teach you a standard process, how to perform proper experiments and collect the necessary amount of data, and how to analyze that data both statistically and graphically to critically interpret the experimental results. An objective decision on the acceptability of any method will depend on being able to define a quality standard for that test. That is perhaps the most critical and often the most difficult judgment that must be made, but once you have that information, the decision on method performance becomes simple and straightforward.

Trends and Directions

The focus here is on the basic process for managing quality and currently available information on quality standards. But of course, things will change and evolve, and you can expect to see new trends and directions.

First, the CLIA criteria for acceptable performance were originally formulated in 1992 and have not been updated since. Expect that the CLIA list of regulated analytes will change, both the analytes on the list and the numerical values for the criteria for acceptable performance. The CLIA regulations include a provision for updating these criteria, but CDC/CMS did not make any changes in the first 15 years. Meanwhile, laboratory testing has moved forward, but there are no CLIA criteria for important tests, such as HbA1c, cTn, and PSA and new tests such as hsCRP. Obviously, changes are needed.

Next, be aware that there are always new management approaches. Management tends to be "trendy," always looking for *New* ways that will bring *New* benefits. The same is true in quality management. Laboratories today may have programs for Total Quality Management, Six Sigma, Lean, Patient Safety, Risk Analysis, and Quality Indicators. They may follow guidelines from CLSI (Clinical Laboratory Standards Institute) and ISO (International Standards Organization). They are subject to inspection from a variety of accreditors, such as CMS (Centers for Medicare and Medicaid Services), CAP (College of American Pathologists), JC (Joint Commission for Accreditation of Healthcare Organizations), and COLA (originally called the Commission for Office Laboratory Accreditation). From my perspective, all these approaches, programs, and guidelines are tools that should be integrated into the basic quality management process described here, rather than being substituted for this basic process.

References

1. Westgard JO, Barry PL. Total quality control: Evolution of quality management systems. Laboratory Medicine 1989;20:377-384.

2. Westgard JO, Barry PL. Beyond quality assurance: Committing to quality improvement. Laboratory Medicine 1989;20:241-247.

3. Westgard JO, Burnett RW, Bowers GN. Quality management science in clinical chemistry: a dynamic framework for continuous improvement of quality. Clin Chem 1990;36:1712-1716.

4. Tonks DB. A study of the accuracy and precision of clinical laboratory determinations in 170 Canadian laboratories. Clin Chem 1963;9:217-233.

5. Barnett RN. Medical significance of laboratory results. Am J Clin Path 1968;50:671-676.

6. 1976 Aspen Conference on Analytical Goals in Clinical Chemistry.

7. Hyltoft Petersen P, Fraser CG, Kallner A, Kenny D. Strategies to set global analytical quality specifications in laboratory medicine. Scand J Clin Lab Invest 1999:59:No.7(Nov).

8. Westgard JO, Hyltoft Petersen P, Wiebe DA. Laboratory process specifications for assuring quality in the U.S. National Cholesterol Education Program. Clin Chem 1991;37:656-661.

9. Westgard JO, Wiebe DA. Cholesterol operational process specifications for assuring the quality required by CLIA proficiency testing. Clin Chem 1991;37:1938-1944.

10. Hyltoft-Petersen P, Ricos C, Stockl D, Libeer J-C, Baadenhuijsen H. Fraser CG, Thienpont L. Proposed guidelines for the internal quality control of analytical results in the medical laboratory. Eur J Clin Chem Clin Biochem 1996;34:983-999.

11. Fraser CG, Hyltoft Petersen P, Ricos C, Haeckel R. Proposed quality specifications for the imprecision and inaccuracy of analytical systems for clinical chemistry. Eur J Clin Chem Clin Biochem 1992;30:311-317.

12. Klee GG. Tolerance limits for short-term analytical bias and analytical imprecision derived from clinical assay specificity. Clin Chem 1993;39:1514-1518.

13. Ricos C, Alvarez V, Cava F, Garcia-Lario JV, Hernandez A, Jimenez CV, Minchinela J, Perich C, Simon M. Current databases on biological variation: pros, cons and progress. Scand J Clin Lab Invest 1999;59:491-500.

14. Fraser C. Biologic Variation: From principles to practice. AACC Press, Washington DC, 2001.

15. Westgard JO. Six Sigma Quality Design and Control: Desirable precision and requisite QC for laboratory testing processes. Second Edition. Madison, WI:Westgard QC, Inc., 2007.

Self-Assessment Questions:

○ What are the 5 components needed to manage quality?

○ Where does method validation fit in this quality management process?

○ Why is method validation important?

○ What drives or guides the quality management process?

3: What is the purpose of a method validation study?

Dr. Westgard reveals the inner, hidden, deeper, secret meaning of method validation. Knowledge of this "meaning" should make the whole method validation process more rational and understandable.

Objectives:

O Understand what method validation studies are supposed to study.

O Recognize the potential shortcoming of statistics in a method validation study.

O Identify the different types of analytical errors that need to be assessed.

Lesson materials:

O **MV – The inner, hidden, deeper, secret meaning,** by James O. Westgard, PhD

Things to do:

O Study the lesson.

O Review a method validation report from the scientific literature.

Method Validation:
The Inner, Hidden, Deeper, Secret Meaning

James O. Westgard, PhD

When I was a freshman in college, I had an English professor who taught me something I've never forgotten. He always asked, "What's the inner, hidden, deeper, secret meaning in what you're writing?" In other words, what are you really trying to accomplish? You'd better figure it out if you expect someone else to understand it. Sure, you can write something, but you've really got to be clear on what you want to accomplish, otherwise the true purpose and meaning will remain a secret.

The real surprise came on my first job as a clinical chemist when I began evaluating the performance of a new multichannel chemistry analyzer. I studied all the existing scientific literature that provided guidelines for performing method validation (MV) studies, but it wasn't at all clear how to tell whether or not a new method was acceptable. No one was telling the secret! And that secret is of paramount importance to evaluate a method properly. Sure, you can collect some data, calculate some statistics, and provide some paper in a folder to show a lab inspector, but is that really why you're doing this?

While I won't claim my English professor made me a better writer (nor can you blame him), he did make me a better scientist by helping me search for the deeper meaning and real purpose in what I do. What's the real purpose of method validation? What's the problem we're trying to solve? Does the present practice provide a correct solution? Is there a better way to do this? How do you know what's the right way to validate the performance of a method?

The Secret Revealed

Here's the inner, hidden, deeper, secret meaning of method validation – and you don't have to read any further to get the message – ERROR ASSESSMENT. You want to estimate how much error might be present in a test result produced by a method in your laboratory. With this information, you then want to be sure that amount of error won't affect the interpretation of the test result and compromise patient care. If your observed errors are so large they can cause an incorrect interpretation, the method isn't acceptable. To be acceptable, the observed errors need to be small relative to changes that will cause a change in the interpretation of a test result.

A focus on analytical errors is the key to the whole method validation process. What kinds of analytical errors might occur with a laboratory method? What experiments can provide data about those errors? What's the best way to perform those experiments to assess the errors? How much data needs to be collected to obtain good estimates of errors? What statistics best estimate the size of those errors from the experimental data? What size errors are allowable without affecting the interpretation of a test and compromising patient care?

Method validation is about error assessment – that's the secret!

A Quick Proof

The correlation coefficient is a statistic that is almost always calculated and reported to describe the results from a comparison of methods study. A value of 1.000 indicates perfect correlation between the results of two methods. Other statistics (such as slope, intercept, and standard deviation of the residuals) can also be calculated from the same data to estimate the size of errors occurring between the methods. Which are more useful?

Consider the following situation. Here's a new cholesterol method where the results from a comparison of methods study give a correlation coefficient of 0.999, which is very close to ideal value of 1.000. Sounds pretty good, doesn't it? How close are the results between the two methods? Is the new method acceptable? Let me give you some additional information.

Here's the plot of the test results by the new method vs those from the comparative method. Note first that the correlation coefficient shows that the results are *close to the best line of fit* between the methods; it does not show that the test values are the *same* as the comparative values.

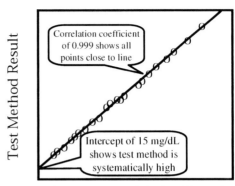

Comparative Method Result

Results of a comparison study, where the new or "test" method values are plotted on y-axis and comparison values on x-axis.

The plot shows that almost all the new method values are systematically higher by 15 mg/dL. Does this information that there is a systematic error of 15 mg/dL help with your decision on the acceptability of the new method? It doesn't look so good anymore, does it? Being in error by 15 mg/dL may limit the usefulness of the test results produced by the new method.

As laboratory people, we intuitively understand errors and have a sense of how they might affect the interpretation of test results and the related care of patients. We don't have the same sense about statistics! That's why statistics should be used to estimate the errors that are meaningful to us[1] – that's a second important secret and we'll deal with it in detail later.

From this simple example, you can recognize the difficulty in interpreting a correlation coefficient, since it doesn't provide a useful estimate of analytical errors. Information about the *size* of analytical errors is more useful for judging the performance of a method[2]. The fact that the correlation coefficient is commonly calculated doesn't make it useful. It just shows that people don't know the secret of method validation!

Analytical Errors

Let's focus on analytical errors and be sure we have a common understanding of the different kinds of errors that need to be estimated. Here's a list of terms that you need to understand: random error or imprecision, systematic error or inaccuracy, constant error, proportional error, and total error.

Random error, RE, or imprecision

Random error is described as an error that can be either positive or negative, whose direction and exact magnitude cannot be predicted, as shown in the accompanying figure by the distribution of results for replicate measurements made on a single specimen.

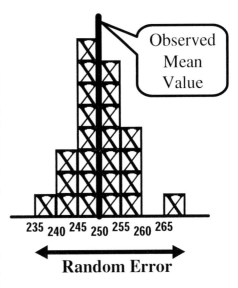

Imprecision is usually quantitated by calculating the standard deviation (SD) from the results of a set of replicate measurements.

Random Error (RE) or Imprecision, as shown by the distribution of test values.

The SD often increases as the concentration increases, therefore it is often useful to calculate the coefficient of variation (CV) to express the SD as a percentage of the mean concentration from the replication study. The maximum size of a random error is commonly expressed as a 2 SD or 3 SD estimate to help understand the potential size of the error that might occur.

Systematic error, SE, or inaccuracy

A systematic error is an error that is always in one direction, as shown in the accompanying figure where a systematic shift displaces the mean of the distribution from its original value. In contrast to random errors that may be either negative or positive and whose direction cannot be predicted, systematic errors are in one direction and cause all the test results to be either high or low.

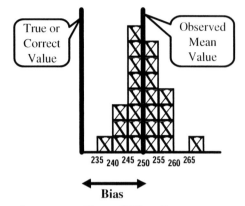

Systematic Error (SE) or Inaccuracy, as shown by shift or bias between mean value and correct value.

How high or how low can be described by the bias, which is calculated as the average difference, or the difference between averages of the values by the "test" method and a "comparative" method in a comparison of methods experiment. Alternatively, the expected systematic difference may be predicted from the equation of the line that best fits the graphical display of test method values on the y-axis vs comparative method values on the x-axis. SE may stay the same over a range of concentrations, in which case it can also be called constant error, or it may change as concentration changes, in which case it can be called proportional error.

Total Error, TE

Total error is the net or combined effect of random and systematic errors, as shown in the accompanying figure. It represents a "worst-case" situation, or just how far wrong a test result might be due to both random and systematic errors. Because laboratories typically only make a single measurement for each test, that measurement can be in error by the expected SE, or bias, plus 2 or 3 SD, depending on how you quantitate the effect of RE.

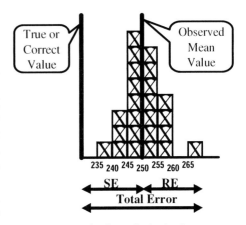

Total Error (TE), includes both systematic error (SE) and random error (RE).

While we in the laboratory like to think about imprecision and inaccuracy as separate errors, the physician and the patient experience the total effect of the two, or the total error. Total error provides a customer or consumer-oriented measure of test performance, which makes it the most important parameter for judging the acceptability of analytical errors.

What's the point?

You must understand the "why" of method validation in order to understand "how" method validation should be accomplished! The "why" defines the purpose, which is to determine the amount of error that might occur with a method. The "how" defines the experimental protocols and data-analysis procedures that provide the estimates of the errors that may occur with the new method. Method validation is all about errors!

Laboratory regulations in the US require that method performance for any new method be "verified" prior to reporting patient test results. **Under the CLIA Final Rule, laboratories must**

verify the reportable range, precision, accuracy, and reference intervals for all *non-waived* methods implemented after April 24, 2003. For methods that are developed in-house or modified by the laboratory, the additional characteristics of analytical sensitivity (detection limit) and analytical specificity (interference, recovery) must also be verified. More extensive reference range studies are also appropriate. The responsibility for method verification or validation, therefore, still resides with each laboratory. While manufacturers will often collect method validation data during the installation of new analytical systems, the laboratory is still accountable to see that adequate data have been collected and that these data show that the new methods provide acceptable performance in the laboratory.

Trends and Directions

Efforts to provide worldwide standards of laboratory practice are going to change the terms and concepts we use. ISO, the International Standards Organization, provides specific guidelines for healthcare laboratories in its document **15189 – Medical Laboratories – Particular requirements for quality and competence** [3]. We will cover this subject in more detail in chapter 21. For now, let's briefly mention what advocates of the ISO approach argue:

"When describing the performance of procedures and the reliability of their results, ISO terminology should be used. Results should be universally comparable and this requires metrological traceability, the concomitant uncertainty indicating reliability should be obtained in a universal and transparent fashion, and should be combinable." [4]

The preferred ISO concepts and terminology are "trueness" and "uncertainty." ***Trueness*** is used to describe the "closeness of agreement between the mean obtained from a large serious of measurements and a true value." This is equivalent to the terms bias and systematic error in this chapter. ***Uncertainty of measurement*** is used by ISO to describe a "parameter, associated with the result of a measurement that characterizes the dispersion of the values that could reasonably be attributed to the measurand," where measurand refers to the particular analyte or test. Uncertainty describes a range of values that correspond to a given test result, e.g., a test result of 200 may have a "standard uncertainty" (SD, CV) of 4 units or 2%, indicating that a value of 200 represents an "expanded uncertainty" of 192 to 208 units (95% or 2SD confidence interval). This concept sounds and looks similar to precision, but the estimate of uncertainty also incorporates any bias or trueness, thus it is actually closer to the idea of total error.

These concepts of trueness and uncertainty come from the world of metrology, where customers are provided with products having assigned target values along with the uncertainty that expresses the correctness or "doubt" in the target value. The ISO approach expects customers to know the meaning of uncertainty. The world of laboratory medicine is different. Physician customers and patient consumers are not necessarily knowledge about the science of measurements and the uncertainty in test results. It would be better if laboratories managed their analytical methods to verify the attainment of the intended clinical quality of results, but in the absence of doing so, it will become necessary to inform the customer of the actual "doubt" of the reported results. Measurement uncertainty is almost certainly part of your future responsibilities.

References

1. Westgard JO, Hunt MR. Use and interpretation of common statistical tests in method comparison studies. Clin Chem 1973;19:49-57.

2. Westgard JO, Carey RN, Wold S. Criteria for judging precision and accuracy in method development and evaluation. Clin Chem 1974;20:825-33.

3. ISO/FDIS 15189 Medical laboratories – Particular requirrements for quality and competence. 2003. International Organization for Standards, Geneva Switz.(Note that a 2nd edition of 15189 was published in 2007 and a 3rd edition is expected to be released by the end of 2008.)

4. Dybkaer R. Setting quality specifications for the future with newer approaches to defining uncertainty in laboratory medicine. Scand J Clin Lab Invest 1999;37:579-584.

Self-Assessment Questions:

○ What are the two major types of analytical errors?

○ What is meant by "total error"?

○ How is total error related to the basic types of errors?

○ How does your literature report describe the errors of the method?

○ What statistics are used in the literature report?

○ How do the report's conclusions relate to the errors of the method?

4: What are the regulatory requirements for method validation?

Dr. Sharon S. Ehrmeyer reviews the US government's CLIA (Clinical Laboratory Improvement Amendments) guidelines that relate method validation requirements to the complexity of the laboratory test. She also describes the method validation requirements of professional accreditation organizations such as the College of American Pathologists (CAP) and the Joint Commission.

Objectives:

○ Classify laboratory tests on the basis of the CLIA complexity guidelines.

○ Relate the complexity classification of a test to the experimental studies required to validate or verify the performance characteristics of a laboratory method.

○ Compare regulatory and accreditation requirements for method validation.

Lesson materials:

○ **MV – The regulations**, by Sharon S. Ehrmeyer, PhD

Things to do:

○ Study the lesson.

○ Access the CLIA website to find the latest test classifications: http://www.cms.gov/clia/

Method Validation:
The Regulations

Sharon S. Ehrmeyer, PhD

Until the Final CLIA Rule was published, many laboratories escaped the requirements to validate the performance of their methods. The February 28, 1992 rules [1] provided an exception for laboratories that performed moderately complex tests using unmodified FDA-approved analytical methods and systems. These sites could accept the manufacturer's performance specifications in lieu of performing method validation studies themselves. All this changed on January 24, 2003 with the issuance of the *Final* CLIA Final Rule [2]. Now ALL non-waived (moderate and high complexity) testing methods require in-lab validation of method performance. CMS provided an "educational" period during which citations were not issued, but as of January 1, 2008, the method validation requirements *must* be met or the laboratory will be cited for deficiencies in this area.

While CLIA sets the *minimum* testing requirements, testing sites can choose to meet the requirements (which may be *more* stringent) of accreditation organizations with CLIA-deemed status, such as the Joint Commission (JC) [3], the College of American Pathologists (CAP) [4], and COLA (formerly the Commission on Office Laboratory Accreditation) [5]. There are also state health laboratory organizations in Washington and New York, which are approved by the government (have exempt status) and impose specific require- ments. In addition, it is always important to keep in mind those practices that would be expected as part of professional responsibility and good laboratory practice.

Quality Systems and the Total Testing Process

The CLIA Final Rule focuses on "quality systems," a new term in this revision. CMS identifies these key components of a quality system:

- General laboratory systems
- Pre-analytic systems
- Analytic systems
- Post-analytic systems

All of these components are important for assuring the quality of laboratory testing services. All must be managed, monitored, and improved. In the CLIA Final Rule, the process of assuring the quality of laboratory testing is called quality assessment, rather than quality assurance or quality management, as it was called in earlier revisions.

Regardless of the terminology chosen, the intent of the Final Rule is to promote the development, implementation, delivery, monitoring, and improvement of high quality laboratory services. This requires an effective quality management system. In this context, *Quality system* refers to the organization, structure, resources, processes, and procedures needed to implement quality management. *Process* means one or more interrelated resources and/or activities that transform inputs into outputs. *Procedure* represents a specified way to perform an activity.

The Final Rule is organized around the flow of a specimen through the laboratory. This path is termed the "total testing process" and includes pre-analytic, analytic, and post-analytic processes and procedures, as shown in the accompanying figure.

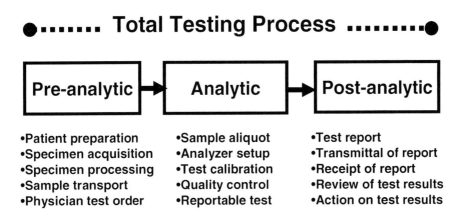

● ······· **Total Testing Process** ········●

| Pre-analytic | → | Analytic | → | Post-analytic |

•Patient preparation
•Specimen acquisition
•Specimen processing
•Sample transport
•Physician test order

•Sample aliquot
•Analyzer setup
•Test calibration
•Quality control
•Reportable test

•Test report
•Transmittal of report
•Receipt of report
•Review of test results
•Action on test results

The term *quality assessment* is used to broadly encompass the practices of measuring and monitoring processes and procedures, including validation and verification, as well as related terms such as evaluation, audit, etc. In our focus on the analytic process, quality assessment should involve sound scientific methodology and data analysis (statistics) to provide an objective comparison of the measured or observed performance to the defined quality goals and requirements.

General requirements for quality control of laboratory tests

Subpart K, Quality Systems for Nonwaived Testing, begins with the following general requirements:

§493.1200 (a) Each laboratory that performs nonwaived testing must establish and maintain written policies and procedures that implement and monitor quality systems for all phases of the total testing process (that is, preanalytic, analytic, and postanalytic), as well as general laboratory systems. (b) The laboratory's quality systems must include a quality assessment component that ensures continuous improvement of the laboratory's performance and services through ongoing monitoring that identifies, evaluates and resolves problems. (c) The various components of the laboratory's quality system are used to meet the requirements in this part and must be appropriate for the specialties and subspecialties of testing the laboratory performs, services it offers, and clients it serves.

§493.1250, Analytic Systems, requires laboratories to meet the requirements for the following:

§493.1251 Procedure manual

§493.1252 Test systems, equipment, instruments, reagents, materials, and supplies

§493.1253 Establishment and verification of method performance specifications

§493.1254 Maintenance and function checks

§493.1255 Calibration and calibration verification procedures

§493.1256 Control procedures

§493.1261-1278 Specialty and subspecialty requirements

§493.1281 Comparison of test results

§493.1282 Corrective actions

§493.1283 Test records

§493.1289 Analytic systems assessment

In this discussion, we consider those requirements for the "establishment and verification of method performance specifications," i.e., method validation, plus comparison of test results and calibration verification.

Method Validation and Test Complexity

The recommendations that must be followed depend on the "complexity" of the test. The CLIA Final Rule combined moderate and high complexity into a Non-Waived classification that governs method validation. Information about classification of specific test methods is available from the CMS website at the address:
http://www.cms.gov/clia/

Waived Tests. The minimum requirement for waived testing under CLIA is to follow the manufacturer's directions. There are no requirements for method validation.

Non-Waived Tests Approved by FDA. Most tests performed in laboratories today fall in this category, thus most method validation studies should follow the recommendations in section §493.1253:

§493.1253 Establishment and verification of performance specifications.

(a) Applicability. Laboratories are not required to verify or establish performance specifications for any test system used by the laboratory before April 24, 2003.

(b)(1) Verification of performance specifications. Each laboratory that introduces an unmodified, FDA-cleared or approved test system must do the following before reporting patient test results:

(i) Demonstrate that it can obtain performance specifications comparable to those established by the manufacturer for the following performance characteristics:

(A) Accuracy.

(B) Precision.

(C) Reportable range of test results for the test system.

(ii) Verify that the manufacturer's reference intervals (normal values) are appropriate for the laboratory's patient population.

This would generally mean performing four experiments:

- Comparison of methods experiment to estimate inaccuracy or bias;
- Replication experiment to estimate imprecision;
- Linearity experiment to determine the reportable range;
- Collecting reference values to verify the reference range. [alternatively, the laboratory medical director can document that the manufacturer's ranges or textbook ranges are appropriate for the clientele being served.]

Non-Waived Tests Modified or Developed In-House. Testing sites that modify moderate complexity tests or use tests developed in-house or tests classified as high complexity under CLIA must follow more stringent method validation requirements, as follows:

§493.1253(b)(2) Each laboratory that modifies an FDA-cleared or approved test system, or introduces a test system not subject to FDA clearance or approval (including methods developed in-house and standardized methods such as textbook procedures, Gram stain, or potassium hydroxide preparations), or uses a test system in which performance specifications are not provided by the manufacturer must, before reporting patient test results, establish for each test system the performance specifications for the following performance characteristics, as applicable:

(i) Accuracy.

(ii) Precision.

(iii) Analytical sensitivity.

(iv) Analytical specificity to include interfering substances.

(v) Reportable range of test results for the test system.

(vi) Reference intervals (normal values).

(vii) Any other performance characteristic required for test performance.

(3) Based upon the performance specifications verified or established in accordance with paragraph (b)(1) or (b)(2) of this section, determine the test system's calibration and control procedures for patient testing as required under §493.1255 and §493.1256.

This would mean performing seven different experiments:

- Comparison of methods experiment to estimate inaccuracy/bias
- Replication experiment to estimate imprecision;
- Linearity experiment to determine reportable range;
- Detection limit experiment to estimate lowest concentration that can be measured;
- Interference experiment to determine constant interferences;
- Recovery experiment to determine proportional intereferences;
- Extensive reference value study to estimate reference range(s).

These experimental studies must be documented. Section §493.1253(c) requires that the laboratory keep the method validation documentation for at least as long as the method is in use.

It is important to note that these requirements are NOT retroactive, meaning that any method in use *prior* to the implementation of the CLIA Final Rule on April 24, 2003 need not be re-verified.

Specific Rules for Calibration and Calibration Verification

Calibration. There are additional requirements for calibration, as follows:

§493.1255 (a) Perform and document calibration procedures –

(1) Following the manufacturer's test system instructions, using calibration materials provided or specified, and with at least the frequency recommended by the manufacturer;

(2) Using criteria verified or established by the laboratory as specified in 493.1253(b)(3) –

(i) Using calibration materials appropriate for the test system and, if possible, traceable to a reference method or reference material of known value;

(ii) Including the number, type, and concentration of calibration materials, as well as acceptable limits for and the frequency of calibration; and

(3) Whenever calibration verification fails to meet the laboratory's acceptable limits for calibration verification.

In short, this means that laboratories must follow the manufacturer's directions for calibration, re-calibrate as frequently as recommended by the manufacturer, plus re-calibrate whenever calibration verification fails.

Calibration verification. This is the process of verifying that calibration remains stable. In many ways, the procedure for doing this is similar to the experiment for reportable range. The specific requirements are as follows:

§493.1255 (b) Perform and document calibration verification procedures -

(1) Following the manufacturer's calibration verification instructions:

(2) Using criteria verified or established by the laboratory under 493.1253(b)(3) –

(i) Including the number, type, and concentration of the materials, as well as acceptable limits for calibration verification; and

(ii) Including at least a minimal (or zero) value, a mid-point value, and a maximum value near the upper limit of the range to verify the laboratory's reportable range of test results for the test system; and

(3) At least once every 6 months and whenever any of the following occur:

(i) A complete change of reagents for a procedure is introduced, unless the laboratory can demonstrate that changing reagent lot numbers does not affect the range used to report patient test results, and control values are not adversely affected by reagent lot number changes.

(ii) There is major preventive maintenance or replacement of critical parts that may influence test performance.

(iii) Control materials reflect an unusual trend or shift, or are outside of the laboratory's acceptable limits, and other means of assessing and correcting unacceptable control values fail to identify and correct the problem.

(iv) The laboratory's established schedule for verifying the reportable range for patient test results requires more frequent calibration verification.

In summary, laboratories must either verify the calibration, or re-calibrate, at least every 6 months, after a change in reagents, after major preventive maintenance, after replacement of any major components, and anytime there is a quality control problem that persists for some time.

Additional Requirements for Periodic Validation

Finally, there are two other requirements that may lead to additional method validation studies for certain tests.

• Ongoing (at least semi-annual) assessment of accuracy is required for any tests that are not evaluated by a proficiency testing program.

§493.1236 Evaluation of proficiency testing performance. (c) At least twice annually, the laboratory must verify the accuracy of the following: (1) Any test or procedure it performs that is not included in subpart I of this part that is or evaluated or scored by a CMS-approved proficiency testing program. (2) Any test or procedure listed in subpart I of this part for which compatible proficiency testing samples are not offered by a CMS-approved proficiency testing program.

- Tests that are performed by multiple analytical systems require periodic comparison, as follows:

  §493.1281 Comparison of test results. (a) If a laboratory performs the same test using different methodologies or instruments, or performs the same test at multiple testing sites, the laboratory must have a system that twice a year evaluates and defines the relationship between test results using different methodologies, instruments, or testing sites.

JC standards for method validation [3]

Waived tests. Prior to 2007, the JC standards included requirements for waived tests, but they no longer impose these requirements. Laboratories can just accept the manufacturer's claims for performance.

Non-Waived (Moderate and High Complexity) Tests Approved by FDA. While JC requires the same general QC requirements as CLIA, JC also has specific method validation requirements (QC.1.70). JC identifies the elements of performance as follows:

- Before a new test, method, or instrument is used to report patient results, the laboratory validates that the test, method, or instrument will consistently produce accurate results.

- The laboratory validates accuracy, precision, and reportable range for an approved unmodified test, method, or instrument for which the manufacturer has established the performance specifications.

- The laboratory establishes performance specifications that include accuracy, precision, analytical sensitivity, analytical specificity, the reportable range, and the reference intervals (normal values) for modified tests, methods, or instruments.

  Note: Modified tests, methods, or instruments include the following:.

  ♦ Test procedures with modifications to the FDA-approved use for specimen type, reagents, instrument, procedural steps, or other components

- ◆ Tests or methods developed in the laboratory with no FDA evaluation

- ◆ Tests, methods, or instruments not subject to FDA clearance

- When a new test, method, or instrument replaces an old test, method, or instrument, correlations are performed between the old test, method or instrument and the new.

  Note: If replacement of the test, method, or instrument is due to poor performance, EP 1 of this standard is followed.

  - ◆ For each new tests, methods, or instruments, the laboratory has made the determination that the reference intervals apply (normal values) to the specific patient population tested.

  - ◆ The laboratory has documented the validation of new tests, methods, or instruments implemented.

  - ◆ The laboratory establishes the number, type, and frequency of quality control materials using the performance specifications verified or established by the laboratory.

  - ◆ Over time the laboratory monitors the accuracy and precision of test performance that may be influenced by changes in test system performance and environmental conditions, and variance in operator performance.

  JC accepts QC data and test performance history as the "evidence" of adequate method performance when a method used in one location is instituted in another location.

CAP's Laboratory Accreditation Program standards for method validation [4]

Waived tests. Like JC, CAP no longer requires method validation for waived testing (see its 9/07 LAB GEN Checklist, page 58). However, a reference range must be identified.

Non-waived tests. CAP's philosophy is that all clinical laboratory testing needs to meet the requirements defined under Section §493.1253(b)(2) of CLIA '88.

The 2007 CAP Checklist GEN (Laboratory General) includes performance specification requirements – accuracy and precision (GEN: 42020), reportable range (GEN: 42085), sensitivity or the lower detection limit (GEN: 42025), and reference range (GEN: 42162) – for each test procedure. Specificity (GEN: 42030) implies an evaluation of the method's ability to respond correctly to the concentration of analyte in the presence of interfering substances. CAP's Checklist now states:

> "Has the laboratory verified or established and documented analytic interferences for each test? Interfering substances pose a significant problem to the clinical laboratory and healthcare providers who may be misled by laboratory results that do not reflect patient clinical status. The laboratory must be aware of common interferences by performing studies or having available studies performed elsewhere (such as by the instrument reagent manufacturer)."

What's the point?

The CLIA Final Rule regulations set *minimum* standards for quality management of testing processes. Other inspection agencies and organizations must provide standards that are *at least as demanding as CLIA* to be approved by CMS for inspection and accreditation of US laboratories. As of 2008, these accreditors have adapted their standards to be consistent with CLIA, in some cases *lowering or eliminating* their earlier requirements.

- For non-waived methods approved by FDA, you must validate the precision, accuracy, reportable range, and reference intervals for any new test or analytic system.

- For non-waived methods NOT approved by FDA or modified by the laboratory, you must validate the additional characteristics of analytical sensitivity and analytical specificity.

- In addition, every six months you must validate the accuracy of methods where an approved proficiency test program is *not* available, compare test results if there are multiple methods in service, and verify calibration whenever there are significant changes in reagents, components, and performance (QC problems).

References

1. U.S. Department of Health and Human Services. Medicare, Medicaid and CLIA programs: Regulations implementing the Clinical Laboratory Improvement Amendments of 1988 (CLIA). Final rule. *Fed Regist* 1992; 57:7002-186.

2. US Centers for Medicare & Medicaid Services (CMS). Medicare, Medicaid, and CLIA Programs: Laboratory Requirements Relating to quality Systems and Certain Personnel Qualifications. Final Rule. Fed Regist Jan 24 2003;16:3640-3714. See also the CMS website http://www.cms.hhs.gov/clia/ and the CMS State Operations Manual Appendix C, Regulations and Interpretive Guidelines for Laboratories and Laboratory Services,
    http://www.cms.hhs.gov/CLIA/
    03_Interpretive_Guidelines_for_Laboratories.asp

3. Accreditation Manual for Pathology and Clinical laboratory Services. Joint Commission (JC). Oakbrook Terrace, IL. 60181

4. CAP Laboratory Accreditation Checklists. College of American Pathologists (CAP). 325 Waukegan Road, Northfield, IL 60093-2750 http://www.cap.org

5. COLA Accreditation Manual. 9881 Broken Land Parkway, Suite 200, Columbia, MD 21046. http://www.cola.org

Self-Assessment Questions

○ What are the test complexity classifications that are used for categorizing the CLIA requirements for method valiation?

○ What are the method validation requirements for waived tests?

○ What are the method validation requirements for non-waived tests approved by the FDA?

○ What are the method validation requirements for non-waived tests not approved by the FDA or modified by the laboratory?

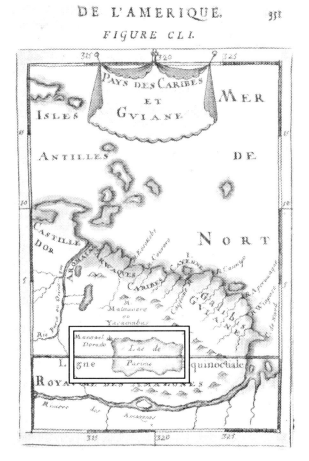

The mythical city of gold: El Dorado!
PAYS des CARIBES et GVIANE, *by Alain Mallet, Paris 1683. The mythical city of gold – Manoeal Dorado – on the western bank of the mythical Lac De Parime.*

Lake Parima and El Dorado (the city of gold) were widely rumored to exist and were well documented on maps of the time, but were never actually implemented (discovered) – much like the US CLIA regulations that described a QC clearance process whose implementation kept being delayed. The Final CLIA Rule (January 24, 2003) made it clear that QC clearance was just a myth. People searched, waited anxiously for new information, and searched some more, but the city of gold never appeared.

5: How is a method selected?

The process of establishing a routine test begins with selection of a method to be evaluated or validated. Dr. Westgard describes different types of method characteristics and identifies those important in method selection and method validation. Example characteristics are included for a cholesterol test.

Objectives:

○ Define the steps in establishing a routine laboratory test.

○ Identify the different types of method characteristics.

○ Recognize the characteristics that are the focus of method validation studies.

Lesson materials:

○ **MV – Selecting a method to validate**,
by James O. Westgard, PhD

Things to do:

○ Study the lesson.

○ Relate the types of characteristics to a common selection problem, such as finding a place to stay, buying a new coat, deciding where to go for dinner, etc.

Method Validation:
Selecting a Method to Validate

James O. Westgard, PhD

Error assessment is what method validation is about, as discussed earlier in *The inner, hidden, deeper, secret meaning.* However, before you can assess any errors, you have to *select* the method to be validated. Method *selection* is a different process that needs to be understood in relation to the validation process that will follow. In fact, there are several processes that are essential for establishing a routine method of analysis.

Establishing a laboratory testing process

Important activities for establishing a routine method of analysis are shown in the accompanying figure. The blocks at the bottom illustrate the key steps involved in routine analysis, where the laboratory acquires specimens, performs tests, checks statistical QC, and reports test results. Those activities are generally regarded as the real work of the laboratory.

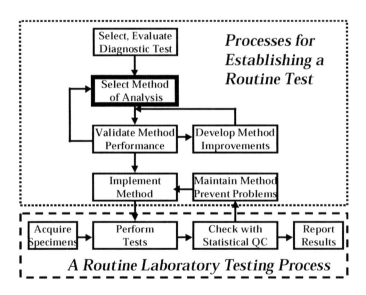

However, for analysis to become routine, the other activities shown in the figure are very important. The selection of the diagnostic test is actually the first step, but this is often skipped for common tests whose medical usefulness is well accepted. For these established tests, we usually start with the selection of the method (the box with the darkest border), then validate its performance. If performance is acceptable, the method is implemented for routine service. If performance is not acceptable, the laboratory may develop some improvements, although that is becoming increasingly difficult with the high degree of automation of many analytical systems. Today it's more likely that a laboratory would select another method rather than attempt to make improvements, then start the validation process over again for the new method.

Once a method has demonstrated acceptable performance, the method must be implemented for routine operation. This involves defining the standard operating procedures and documenting the procedure, selecting an appropriate QC procedure for monitoring routine performance, and training personnel to operate the new method. While in routine service, problems will undoubtedly be identified through QC, which will lead to preventive maintenance procedures to minimize or eliminate those problems. Routine operation is often the simplest part of this overall process **if** the laboratory does a good job of selecting the method, validates method performance, implements the method through careful and thorough in-service training, monitors method performance with a QC procedure that has a low false rejection rate and appropriate error detection, and aggressively maintains the method to identify problems, eliminate sources of error, and prevent future problems.

Method characteristics

The aim when selecting a method is to choose the method that has the best chance of achieving the laboratory's service requirements. The process of selection consists of defining those requirements, searching the technical literature to find information about available methods, then selecting the method whose characteristics best satisfy the laboratory's service requirements.

Careful definition of the requirements is essential [1]. If this step is overlooked, the laboratory may spend considerable time and effort evaluating a method that will not be satisfactory, regardless of method performance. An example might be a point-of-care method that turns out to be too expensive even though its analytical performance is acceptable. Cost should be considered out-front when selecting the method to be evaluated, not after validating method performance.

What characteristics of a method are important? In general, they can be divided into three categories.

- **Application characteristics** are factors that determine whether a method can be implemented in a particular laboratory situation. They consist of cost-per-test, types of specimens that can be analyzed, sample volume, turnaround time, workload, equipment and personnel requirements, space, portability, and safety considerations.

- **Methodology characteristics** are factors which, in principle, should contribute to best performance. In general, these are concerned with the analytical sensitivity and analytical specificity of the method of analysis. They consider the choice of chemical reaction, optimization of reaction conditions, principles of standardization and calibration, and the rigor of the analytical procedure.

- **Performance characteristics** are factors which, in practice, demonstrate how well a method performs. These include the reportable range, precision, recovery, interference, accuracy, and sometimes detection limit.

Let's start with a non-laboratory example to illustrate these different kinds of characteristics. Assume you're selecting a new motorized vehicle.

- **Application characteristics** include your expected use, type of vehicle, price range, body style, color, etc. Your expected use will help define the type of vehicle – tractor, truck, car, or motorbike. Assuming it's a vehicle that will be used to go to work, let's look for a car. If your favorite color is red, you don't have to try out a black car – you can tell by looking whether it satisfies this application characteristic.

- **Methodology characteristics** can be illustrated by the following. If you live in Wisconsin, or worse yet Minnesota (no offense – I've lived there and still visit often), you might want a car with good traction for the winter weather. A four-wheel drive vehicle would be expected to perform better than two-wheel drive. If good mileage were also important, a four-cylinder engine would be a better characteristic than a six or eight cylinder engine. Both four-wheel drive and number of cylinders (or engine size) are methodology characteristics that should help satisfy your performance needs.

- **Performance characteristics** are those factors that you can evaluate by driving the vehicle. Standard measures of performance are acceleration, handling, ride, braking, and mileage. Special measures might include off-road or winter-weather traction. You don't test-drive an expensive, large, black, eight-cylinder, two-wheel drive truck because that vehicle doesn't satisfy your application and methodology characteristics.

Cholesterol example

General characteristics to be considered are the following:

- **Application characteristics** should include the type of specimen, volume of specimen, workload appropriate for the testing situation (high volume centralized lab vs low volume point-of-care), cost per test, time for analysis, operator skills, and operator training requirements.

- **Methodology characteristics** should include the type of standards or calibrators, traceability of standard or calibrator assigned values, chemical principle, reagents and reaction conditions, measurement principle, and measurement capabilities.

- **Performance characteristics** should include the reportable range, imprecision, bias vs the Abell-Kendahl reference method [3], interference, and total errors less than 10%.

High volume automated laboratory characteristics can be defined more specifically:

- **Application characteristics** are serum samples, sample size of less than 10 microliters, test throughput of 200 per hour, cost less than $0.25 per "click" or $0.50 per test.

- **Methodology characteristics** are enzymatic cholesterol esterase reaction, calibrators traceable to the national Abell-Kendahl reference method [3], and accuracy verified by comparison of results with a reference lipid laboratory.

- **Performance characteristics** are a reportable range from 50 to 500 mg/dL, allowable total error of 10% at a concentration of 200 mg/dL, method CV of 3% or less, method bias of 3% or less, no interference with up to 10 mg/dL bilirubin, no interference with lipemia of up to 600 mg/dL triglycerides, and minimal interference from hemolysis.

Point-of-care (POC) characteristics might be quite different, particularly the application characteristics that must take into account the POC setting:

- **Application characteristics** are a whole blood specimen from fingerstick or heparinized sample, turnaround time of 10 minutes or less, ease of use for operators who are not trained in laboratory testing, minimal maintenance and downtime, works or doesn't work operation, cost less than $4.00 per test, impossible to use non-calibrated reagent lot, small, lightweight, and portable.

- **Methodology characteristics** are enzymatic cholesterol esterase reaction, calibration built into test system by manufacturer with lot-specific values traceable to Abell-Kendahl reference method [3], and accuracy verified by comparison of results with a reference lipid laboratory.

- **Performance characteristics** are a reportable range from 100 to 400 mg/dL, allowable total error of 10% at a concentration of 200 mg/dL, no interference with hematocrits up to 55%, no interference from bilirubin up to 5 mg/dL, no interference from lipemia up to 600 mg/dL triglycerides, and minimal interference from hemolysis.

Selection of multi-test analytic systems

It gets much more complicated when trying to select an analytic system that performs many different tests. Analytic systems today can offer a hundred different tests. These are huge instruments that can consolidate much of the laboratory's work onto a single "box." When the objective is consolidation, then application characteristics will dominate the selection process. Methodology characteristics may be of interest for some critical tests, but the analytic quality of many tests will be *assumed* to be acceptable. Nonetheless, every test must be validated for reportable range, precision, accuracy, and reference limits.

As an example of application characteristics in the "real world," a poster presentation [4] at a national meeting focused on the following characteristics: number of different tests available, tests/hour throughput, number of reagents onboard, reagent loading, sample load capacity, sample volume, minimum dead volume, clot/bubble detection, analysis time, lag time after startup, time to first result, STAT capability and time, hours of daily maintenance, onboard maintenance log, software friendliness, QC rules available, and training time. These are complex application characteristics that require careful and thorough study to compare the features of different systems.

Finding all the information is a challenge. Manufacturers often provide descriptions of their analytic systems on their website and in their marketing materials. Comparison of the characteristics of different analytic systems is greatly aided by "instrument comparison reports," such as provided in *CAP Today* from the College of American Pathologists. There are huge exhibits of equipment and systems at national professional meetings, such as the American Association of Clinical Chemistry. Finally, and perhaps most important before the final buying decision, there should be visits to laboratories where the systems are already installed and working.

Information and specifications for method performance may be more difficult to find. While manufacturers are required to make claims for performance to obtain marketing approval from FDA, those performance claims may be difficult to find in their marketing materials. Sometimes method validation studies are published in the scientific literature, but that is usually limited to new tests and new systems. It's more common to find good scientific information in the abstracts and posters presented at professional meetings. For analytic systems that have some history in the field, their comparative performance may be assessed from reports of proficiency testing surveys from organizations such as the College of American Pathologists (CAP), Medical Laboratory Evaluation (MLE), and the American Association of Bioanalysts (AAB).

What's the point?

The selection of a method or analytic system directly leads to the quality of the tests available from a laboratory. Therefore, the selection process itself should be objective and account for the application and methodology characteristics that are important in your laboratory. The selection process is particularly complicated for multi-test analytic systems, where the application characteristics will dominate the decision. To keep analytic quality alive in the decision process, it may be necessary to go beyond consideration of methodology characteristics and look at the comparative performance of methods, as available in survey reports from proficiency testing or external quality assessment programs. The laboratory must validate the performance characteristics of all the tests on the system. And the laboratory will own the quality that it buys.

References:

1. Westgard JO, deVos DJ, Hunt MR, Quam EF, Carey RN, Garber CC. Concepts and practices in the evaluation of laboratory methods. I. Background and Approach. Am J Med Technol 1978;44:290-300.

2. Wiebe DA, Westgard JO. Cholesterol - a model system to relate medical needs with analytical performance. Clin Chem 1993;39:1504-1513.

3. Cooper GR, Smith SJ, Duncan IW, et al. Interlaboratory testing of the transferability of a candidate reference method for total cholesterol in serum. Clin Chem 1986;32:921-929.

4. Perkins SL, Bookalam S, Warr M, Ooi DS. Evaluation of the Architect i1000SR Immunoassay Analyzer. Abstract D-81. Clin Chem 2007/53:A185.

Self-Assessment Questions:

○ What are the three types of method characteristics?

○ Give three examples for each type of method characteristic.

○ Which characteristics are of most interest in method selection?

○ Which characteristics are of most interest in method validation?

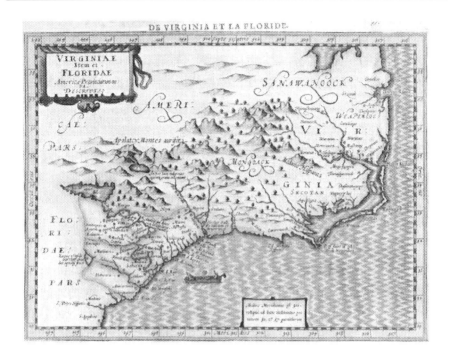

A selection problem!
VIRGINIAE ITEM et FLORIDAE, *by Johannes Cloppenburg, Amsterdam, 1630.*

This map of the southeast coast of the US was prepared from parts of two earlier maps – one of Florida and one of Virginia. While the map was well-executed, i.e., beautifully engraved, it wasn't very useful because it overlooked an important characteristic – the Carolinas. As a result, the "cape islands" at the west side of the Virginia map were brought together with the eastern geography of Florida, without leaving room for the Carolinas. One notorious myth originating with this map is the non-existent lake in the Appalachian Mountains, which became known as Lake Appalachia.

6: What experiments are necessary to validate method performance?

Dr. Westgard explains how to develop an experimental plan for a method validation study. Specific experiments can be used to estimate the magnitude of the different types of analytical errors. These experiments can be organized into a practical plan on the basis of time and effort needed to carry out the different experiments.

Objectives:

- ○ Identify the different experiments used in a method validation study.
- ○ Relate those experiments to the types of errors estimated.
- ○ Organize those experiments into a practical plan for carrying out the study.

Lesson materials:

- ○ **MV – The experimental plan,** by James O. Westgard, PhD

Things to do:

- ○ Study the lesson.
- ○ Review a literature report and its experimental procedures.

Method Validation:
The Experimental Plan

James O. Westgard, PhD

I start this discussion with the assumption that the method to be tested has been carefully selected, as discussed earlier in *Selecting a method to validate*. Therefore, the application requirements have been satisfied and the methodology characteristics have been considered.

We can now focus on the performance characteristics, which include precision, accuracy, interference, reportable range, and sometimes detection limit. These characteristics may already have been estimated by the manufacturer (claims made for the method) or by a user (published in a validation study). These claims or published results still need to be verified to show that the method works properly and is acceptable in *your* particular laboratory. That's the purpose of the method validation study.

Approach for formulating a plan

To carry out a good method validation study, you need to do the following:

- define a quality requirement for the test in the form of the amount of error that is allowable, preferably an allowable total error,
- select appropriate experiments to reveal the expected types of analytical errors,
- collect the necessary experimental data,
- perform statistical calculations on the data to estimate the size of analytical errors,
- compare the observed errors with the defined allowable error, and
- judge the acceptability of the observed method performance.

An experimental plan can be formulated by:

- recognizing the types of errors that need to be assessed for this test and method,
- identifying the appropriate experiments and the amount of data needed to estimate those types of errors, then
- organizing these experiments to perform the quick and easy ones first and the ones taking more time and effort last.

Types of errors to be assessed

All measurements have some error! Even simple measurement devices, such as a bathroom scale, have errors. Whenever you weigh yourself on a bathroom scale, you observe error. That's why you immediately step off the scale, get back on, and make another measurement. You usually observe that these measurements, though performed closely in time and under essentially identical conditions, are still not exactly the same – that's the random error or imprecision discussed earlier in *The inner, secret, deeper, hidden meaning.* You may also have noticed that virtually all scales are inaccurate – they read too high, don't they! That's an example of the systematic error or bias described earlier.

In response to the weight being too high, we usually try to adjust the zero point of the scale and make the results lower. This assumes that there is a systematic error that is constant in nature, i.e., all people who weigh on that scale would be high by the same amount. If instead the weights of all people are in error by a proportion of their total weight, i.e., proportional error, the measurement needs to be corrected by a calibration type of adjustment, rather than a zero point adjustment.

If such simple devices as scales are subject to errors, it is readily understandable that measurements from the complex devices and systems used for laboratory tests are subject to these same kinds of error:

- imprecision or random errors,
- inaccuracy, bias, or systematic errors, which can be of two types
  - constant systematic error or
  - proportional systematic error.

All these errors can be recognized when a group of measurements are compared to the correct or true values. For example, the accompanying figure shows how different types of errors are revealed when the results from a test method are plotted on the y-axis versus those from a comparative method on the x-axis. The dashed line in the middle of the figure represents ideal method

Comparative Method Result

performance where the test method and the comparative method give exactly the same results. The bottom line in the figure shows the effect of a proportional systematic error, where the magnitude of the error increases as the test result gets higher. The top line shows the effect of a constant systematic error, where the whole line is shifted up and all results are high by the same amount. Note that these results will also be subject to the random error of the method, therefore the actual data points would scatter about the line as illustrated in the figure. The range of this scatter above and below the line provides some idea of the amount of random error that is present.

Experiments for estimating analytical errors

While a comparison of methods experiment can reveal all these different types of errors, it is not necessarily the best way to go about studying a new method. For example, random error might be estimated more quickly by simply analyzing a single specimen or a stable control material.

There are specific experiments for estimating different types of analytical errors, as shown in the accompanying table. The first column lists the type of error. The second column is labeled "prelimi-nary" because these experiments are generally easier to perform and take less time and effort than the "final" experiments. The final experiments are more demanding and should be performed after preliminary results have shown that everything was acceptable thus far. However, a poor showing on a preliminary experiment can be grounds for stopping the study and rejecting a method because a specific error condition has been identified.

Type of Analytic Error	Evaluation Experiment	
	Preliminary	Final
Random Error	Replication Within run	Replication Between runs
Constant Error	Interference	Comparison of Methods
Proportional Error	Recovery	

Here's a brief description of these different experiments:

- A **replication experiment** provides information about random error and is performed by making measurements on a series of aliquots of the same test samples within a specified period of time, usually within an analytical run, within a day, or over a period of a month. The preliminary experiment usually involves determining within-run imprecision. The final experiment generally requires at least 20 working days to provide a good estimate of the total imprecision, which includes within- and between-run components.

- An **interference experiment** provides information about the constant systematic error caused by the lack of specificity of the method. One test sample is prepared by adding the suspected material to a sample containing the analyte. A second aliquot of the original sample is diluted by the same amount with solvent, then both samples are analyzed by the test method and the difference determined.

- A **recovery experiment** provides information about the proportional systematic error caused by a competitive reaction. A test sample is prepared by adding a standard solution of the analyte being tested to an aliquot of a patient specimen. A baseline sample is prepared by adding an equal amount of the solvent used for the standard solution to a second aliquot of the same patient specimen. The two samples are then analyzed by the test method and the amount recovered is compared to the amount added.

• A **comparison of methods experiment** is primarily used to estimate the average systematic error observed with real patient samples, but can also reveal the constant or proportional nature of that error. A series of patient specimens are collected and analyzed by both the test method and a comparative analytical method. The results are compared to determine the differences between the methods, which are the analytical errors between the methods.

Organizing the experiments into a plan

A general plan for validating the performance of a new method is outlined below. It includes four phases – the initial familiarization with the method, the "quick and dirty" preliminary evaluation experiments, followed by the more extensive studies of precision and accuracy, and concluding with the steps to implement the method for routine service.

Familiarization period
- Establish working procedure
- Validate reportable range
- Check calibration
- Check detection limit

Preliminary MV experiments
- Perform within-run replication study
- Perform interference study
- Perform recovery study
- Judge analytical acceptability

Final MV experiments
- Perform total replication study
- Perform comparison of methods study
- Judge analytical acceptability
- Verify reference interval(s)
- Document studies

Implementation
- Select QC procedure
- Write operating protocol or procedure
- Train analysts
- Introduce method for service
- Monitor routine performance

Note that this plan can and should be adjusted to consider any unique characteristics of a method or any special requirements of a laboratory and the patients it serves. For example, the studies for interference and recovery might be more extensive if the hospital is a cancer center whose patients are likely being treated with many different drugs. In a transplant center, comparison of methods studies may focus on the transplant patients who are treated with anti-rejection medications. The amount of data collected can also be adjusted on the basis of what's already available in the literature or what's required by regulatory or accreditation guidelines. For example, this plan should take into account the complexity of methods, as classified under the CLIA Final Rule guidelines. Any method developed in-house or any modified manufacturer's method requires more careful study and might apply the CLSI protocols for the replication experiment [1] and the comparison of methods experiments [2]. Unmodified non-waived methods may be tested with simpler experiments that require less time and effort and also less data. For non-waived non-modified FDA-approved methods, there is a simpler protocol [3] intended for user validation of trueness and precision in the laboratory, which will be discussed in chapter 19.

Walking tour of the plan

The first step with any new method is to get the method working and establish an operating protocol. This is the "familiarization" period, where the objective is to learn how to perform the method properly and establish an operating protocol that provides consistent test results. With our bathroom scale, for example, you have to get the scale out of the box, transport it to the proper location, find space to put it, and try it out. With a new analytical method, you have to set up the instrument, prepare the reagents, calibrate the methods, and obtain results from test samples. One of the critical factors is to check the standards and confirm that the method is properly calibrated, otherwise calibration errors will show up throughout the experimental studies.

Once the method is operating, the next step is to determine the reportable range. With our bathroom scale, we generally are concerned that the range be adequate for the weight of a small child to a moderately large adult. The common scale is not likely to be sensitive enough to weigh a small baby, so if a very low detection limit is important, this characteristic needs to be dealt with up-front when selecting the scale. The common scale is also unlikely to handle a 300+ pound football player, so if an extremely wide working range is important, that characteristic again should have been considered during the selection process. Likewise, with a new analytical method, the reportable range will vary from test to test and must be defined as part of the specifications for the method, then checked by analyzing a series of solutions, usually in duplicate or triplicate, whose concentrations cover the range of interest. If detection limit is a critical characteristic, it may be assessed at this time or in the next phase of preliminary experiments.

Next the preliminary experiments would be performed to determine within-run imprecision, recovery, and interference. Minimum amounts of data are collected in the minimum amount of time to facilitate a quick judgment of the acceptability of performance under the simplest conditions. The replication experiment might include 20 samples of two or three materials whose concentrations closely match the medical decision levels of interest for the tests. Interference experiments should test common problems such as hemolysis, lipemia, and high bilirubin. Recovery experiments assess whether there are any competitive reactions due to the matrix or other materials in the native specimens. If the errors revealed by the preliminary experiments are small, the final replication and comparison of methods experiments should be performed.

This final replication experiment should cover at least 20 working days. The comparison of methods experiment will usually be performed on fresh patient specimens, but stored specimens should also be tested if those storage conditions represent the typical processing and handling of the specimens routinely analyzed. The comparative method should ideally be one that has been previously studied and a minimum of 40 well-chosen patient samples should be tested over a minimum of 5 working days. These samples should be distributed one-third in the low to low-normal range, one-third in the normal range, and one-third in the high abnormal range. Once these data have been collected, method acceptability should be judged on the basis of the sizes of the random, systematic, and total analytical errors. If these errors are small compared to the amount of error that would invalidate the use and interpretation of a test result, the method is acceptable. If too large, these errors will make it necessary to reject the method or to identify and eliminate the causes of the errors.

When method performance is judged acceptable, it may still be necessary to estimate or at least verify the reference interval(s). If the performance of the comparative method is not well documented, it may also be necessary to perform clinical studies to correlate test results with clinical conditions. Finally, all these studies need to be documented for future reference.

Implementation starts by writing the method protocol or laboratory procedure, which will be used in training other analysts to perform the new method. An essential part is a description of the quality control procedures that will be used to monitor routine performance. Once analysts are trained and the method is in routine service, it will be very important to monitor performance closely during the first month, identify the sources of problems, improve the preventive maintenance procedures, and update analysts about how to better manage the quality of the method.

What to do?

To perform a method validation study, you need to understand the experiments and organize them into an efficient plan. The outline here provides a starting point, but it can and should be modified for your particular applications. You should write up your plan, complete with procedures that describe the numbers and sources of samples, as well as worksheets for recording the data. It is important to keep on top of the data as it is being collected in order to identify problems as the experiments are being performed. This generally means tabulating and graphing the data prior to statistical analysis. And the problems of interest are both those with the experiments and those with the method! You should draw conclusions about the acceptability of performance as you complete each individual experiment. In the end, the final decision should be based on the maximum or total error expected from the experiments for long-term precision and comparison of methods. Even when the method is judged acceptable, the work is not finished. Implementation requires design of an appropriate QC procedure, documentation of the standard operating procedure, and thorough training of all operators. Method validation is not over until the method demonstrates stable performance under routine operating conditions.

References:

1. CLSI EP5-A2. Evaluation of precision performance of quantitative measurement methods. Approved Guideline 2004. Clinical and Laboratory Standards Institute, Wayne PA.

2. CLSI EP9-A2. Method comparison and bias estimation using patient samples. Approved Guideline 2002. Clinical and Laboratory Standards Institute, Wayne PA.

3. CLSI EP15-A2. User verification of performance for precision and trueness. Approved Guideline 2006. Clinical and Laboratory Standards Institute, Wayne PA.

Self-Assessment Questions:

O   What experiment is used to estimate the imprecision of a method?

O   What experiments are used to estimate the inaccuracy of a method?

O   Why is the reportable range experiment performed early in a study?

O   Why are two different replication experiments usually performed?

O   What's the difference between constant and proportional systematic error?

O   What experiments are used to estimate constant and proportional errors?

7: How are the experimental data analyzed?

Before explaining the details of specific experiments, Dr. Westgard gives an overview of the data analyses that are useful and appropriate for the different experiments. The approach here is to consider data analysis "tools," rather than statistics and equations. These tools are readily available in the form of calculators, electronic spreadsheets, and computer programs. Online calculators are introduced to provide easy-to-use tools for use with this book.

Objectives:

○ Minimize your fear of statistics.

○ Identify the tools and techniques needed for data analysis.

○ Match the tools with the experiments and errors to be estimated.

○ Recognize the capability of available calculation tools.

Lesson materials:

○ **MV – The data analysis tool kit,** by James O. Westgard, PhD

○ **The method validation data analysis tool kit,** http://www.westgard.com/mvtools.html

Things to do:

○ Study the lesson.

○ Practice using the online calculators with the sample data.

○ Review the statistics presented in a published validation report.

Method Validation:
The Data Analysis Tool Kit

James O. Westgard, PhD

This chapter is actually about statistics, but I didn't put "statistics" in the title because too many people get turned off as soon as they see that word. Others become uncomfortable when they see the equations for the statistical calculations. By now – three sentences into this chapter – you may be wondering if you can just skip the chapter and avoid the topic. The answer is NO. You need statistics to make sense of the data collected in method validation experiments.

Tools, not equations!

To reduce the mental roadblocks in understanding statistics, **there aren't any equations in this chapter**. Instead, we're going to assume the calculations can be easily performed with the calculator and computer technology that's available today. Your main job will be to recognize *what* calculations are useful for different sets of data.

When I lecture on this topic, I begin by showing the class a bunch of tools, such as a hammer, wrench, saw, and screwdriver. Office tools (such as a stapler, scissors, paper, and pen) would also provide good examples, but you're too comfortable with those tools. I want you to learn that you can use tools, even if you're not so comfortable with them. So, let's consider the hammer, wrench, saw, and screwdriver.

- Which tool would be most useful for hanging a picture on the wall?

- Which tool would you use to tighten the bows on your sunglasses?

- Which tool do you want to take along at Christmas time when you go into the forest to get your tree?

- Which tool do you hope to have along if your car has a flat tire?

You don't have to be an engineer, mechanic, or carpenter to recognize which tool fits these jobs. Everyone makes use of these tools to do certain basic jobs. While there are more complicated applications that take more skill and knowledge – and sometimes more specialized tools – everyone is capable to making practical use of the common tools.

It can be the same with statistics!

Recommended tools for data analysis

Statistics are just tools for combining many experimental results, i.e., data, and summarizing all that data in just a few numbers. Remember that the objective of each experiment is to estimate the amount of error from the data collected. The key with the statistics is to know which ones will provide useful information about the errors of interest in the different experiments.

Before trying to estimate these errors, we need to define the usable analytical range (or reportable range) of the method so that the experiments can be properly planned and valid data can be collected. The reportable range is usually defined as the range where the analytical response of the method is linear with respect to the concentration of the analyte being measured.

Then we start the error analysis. First, we want to know the imprecision or random error from the 20 or more data points collected in a replication experiment. Then we need to estimate the systematic error from the 40 or more data points collected in a comparison of methods experiment. Finally, we need to make a judgment on the performance of the method on the basis of the errors that have been observed. The statistics are used to make reliable estimates of the errors from the data that have been collected.

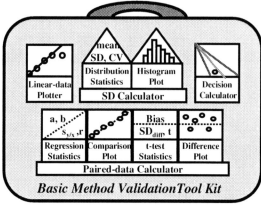

Basic Method Validation Tool Kit

Here's a picture of the tool kit you need to analyze the data from basic method validation experiments. The tool kit includes several calculators and plotters:

- **Linear-data plotter** to display the observed method response versus the relative or assigned concentrations for a series of solutions or specimens;

- **SD calculator** to determine distribution statistics (mean, SD, CV) and to display a histogram of the distribution;

- **Paired-data calculator** to determine regression statistics (slope or a, y-intercept or b, standard deviation about the regression line or $s_{y/x}$, and correlation coefficient, r), display the data in a "comparison plot" (test method as y, comparison method as x), determine t-test statistics (bias, SD_{diff}, t-value), and display data in a difference plot (y-x vs x);

- **Decision calculator** to judge performance.

Note that these tools often include both calculations and graphical displays of the data. There is an association between certain calculations and graphs because they complement each other for describing and displaying a set of data. For example, distribution statistics are used with a histogram plot to describe and display data for imprecision or random error. For inaccuracy or systematic error, regression statistics are used with a comparison plot, or t-test statistics are used with a difference plot.

Note also that there is a natural order for using the tools, as suggested by their location in the tool kit. Those at the top are generally pulled out first, e.g., the linear-data plotter is used in the beginning to establish the reportable range of the method, after which the SD calculator will be used to estimate the imprecision or random error, whose acceptability can be assessed using the decision calculator. After these steps, the paired-data calculator will be used to estimate the inaccuracy of the method and the decision calculator used again to assess the overall performance of the method.

Where to get the tools

These calculator tools may be obtained from handheld calculators (e.g., Texas Instruments), electronic spreadsheets (e.g., Excel), common statistics packages (Minitab, SAS, SPSS), specialized method validation software written for laboratory applications, and also from the online calculators on Westgard Web. Many of these sources will also provide appropriate graphical displays, or you can construct them manually using graph paper. The Method Decision Chart can very easily be constructed manually with graph paper.

Chapter 8 provides more information about the calculations. Later chapters provide more detailed discussion about the use and interpretation of statistics with individual experiments. For now we're going to focus on the bigger picture – which tools are appropriate for the different method validation experiments.

When to use each tool

Given a set of experimental data, you need to recognize which tool is right for that job. Here are some general guidelines:

- **Random error (RE)** is almost always estimated by calculating a standard deviation. The experiment itself determines which factors contribute to the estimate, e.g., the replication experiment limits the RE to just the method being tested, whereas the comparison of methods experiment can provide an estimate of the RE between methods, which depends on the variation observed for both the test and comparison method.

- **Systematic error (SE)** is related in some way to the calculation of a mean or average. This may be the average difference between paired samples in a comparison of methods study, or the difference between the means between two methods, or a representation of the average relationship as given by the line of best fit through the method comparison data.

- Remember that a decision on the **acceptability** of a method's performance is a judgment on whether the observed errors will affect the medical usefulness of the test. The statistics provide the best estimate of the size of the errors [1]. You have to make the judgment on whether those errors will affect the medical usefulness of the test [2]. You can do this by defining a quality requirement in the form of an allowable total error, TE_a, such as defined by the CLIA proficiency testing criteria for acceptable performance. A simple graphical tool called the Method Decision Chart can be used to help you judge method performance [3].

Example tools for educational use

Online calculators for educational use are available on Westgard Web at **http://www.westgard.com/mvtools.html**. These web-tools should be useful for working with example data sets and problem sets. However, they are not intended to answer all your data analysis needs for method validation studies. It is also recommended that you acquire your own calculator tools, either a general statistics program, a specialized method validation program, or an electronic spreadsheet.

The linear-data plotter is used with the data collected in the linearity experiment, where the purpose is to assess the analytical range over which patient results may be reported. The response of the method is plotted on the y-axis versus the relative concentration or assigned values of the samples or specimens on the x-axis. The "reportable range" is generally estimated as the linear working range of the analytical method.

The SD calculator is used for the data collected in the replication experiment, where the objective is to estimate the random error or imprecision of the method on the basis of repeated measurements on the same sample material. The statistics that should be calculated are the mean, SD, and CV. Also be sure to record the number of measurements used in the calculations.

- The mean, or average of the group of results, describes the central location of the measurements.

- The SD describes the expected distribution of results, i.e., 66% are expected to be within ± 1 SD of the mean, 95% within ± 2 SD of the mean, and 99.7% within ± 3 SD of the mean.

- The CV, or coefficient of variation, is equal to the SD divided by the mean, multiplied by 100 to express in percent.

- The histogram displays the distribution of results. Ideally, the distribution should appear Gaussian, or "normal."

The paired data calculator may be used with the pairs of results on each specimen analyzed by the test and comparison methods in the comparison of methods experiment. This is the most complicated part of the statistical analysis and requires the most care and attention. Linear regression statistics may be used with a comparison plot, or t-test statistics may be used along a difference plot.

The regression statistics that should be calculated are the slope (b) and y-intercept of the line (a), the standard deviation of the points about that line ($s_{y/x}$), and the correlation coefficient (r, the Pearson product moment correlation coefficient). You may also see the slope designated as m, the y-intercept as b, and the standard deviation as $s_{residuals}$, respectively. The correlation coefficient is included to help you decide whether the linear regression statistics or the t-test statistics will provide the most reliable estimates of systematic error.

- The slope describes the angle of the line that provides the best fit to the test and comparison results. A perfect slope would be 1.00. Deviations from 1.00 are an indication of proportional systematic error [1].

- The y-intercept describes where the line of best fit intersects with the y-axis. Ideally, the y-intercept should be 0.0. Deviations from 0.0 are an indication of constant systematic error [1].

- The $s_{y/x}$ term describes the scatter of the data around the line of best fit. It provides an estimate of the random error *between methods* which includes both the imprecision of the test and comparison methods, as well as possible matrix effects that vary from one specimen to another. It will never be zero because both the test and comparison methods have some imprecision [1].

- The correlation coefficient describes how well the results between the two methods change together. An r of +1.00 indicates perfect correlation, i.e., all the points fall perfectly on a line that shows the test method values vs the comparison method values. Values less than 1.00 indicate there is scatter in the data about the line of best fit. The lower the r value, the more scatter in the data. The main use of r is to help you assess the reliability of the linear regression calculations – **r should never be used as an indicator of method acceptability** [1]. When r is 0.99 or greater, linear regression calculations will provide reliable estimates of errors. When r is less than 0.975, it is better to use the paired data calculations or an alternate (and more complicated) regression technique such as Deming or Passing-Bablock regression [4,5].

- A comparison plot should be used to display the data from the comparison of methods experiment (plotting the comparison method value on the x-axis and the test method value on the y-axis). This plot is then used to visually inspect the data to identify possible outliers and to assess the range of linear agreement [1].

The t-test statistics of interest are the bias, SD of the differences, and lastly, something called a t-value which also requires knowledge of the number of paired sample measurements. Again, be sure to keep track of the number of measurements, which for the comparison of methods experiment is the number of patient specimens compared.

- The bias is the difference between the averages by the two methods, which is also the same as the average difference for all the specimens analyzed by the two methods. It provides an estimate of the systematic error or average difference that is expected between the methods – the smaller the bias, the smaller the systematic error, the better the agreement.

- The SD of the differences provides an estimate of the random error between the methods. It will never be zero because both the test and comparison methods have some imprecision.

- The t-value itself is an indicator of whether enough paired sample measurements have been collected to know whether the observed bias is real, or statistically significant. As a rule of thumb, in a method comparison experiment where the minimum of 40 patient specimens have been compared, if t is greater than 2.0, the data is sufficient to conclude that a bias exists. It's important to note that it's the size of the bias that's important in judging the acceptability of the method, not the size of the t-value.

- A difference plot should be used to display the differences between paired results, plotting the difference between the test method minus comparison method values on the y-axis versus the comparison method result on the x-axis. Difference plots are popular today because of their simplicity [6], however, their use and interpretation are not so simple when you want to make a quantitative, objective decision about performance [7].

The decision calculator is used to display the estimates of random and systematic errors and judge the performance of the method [3]. Therefore, this chart depends on the estimates of errors that are obtained from other statistical calculations. In brief, the chart is drawn on the basis of the quality requirement that is defined for the method and shows the allowable inaccuracy on the y-axis versus the allowable imprecision on the x-axis. The observed imprecision and inaccuracy of the method are then plotted to display the method's "operating point" (y-coordinate is the estimate of inaccuracy or SE, x-coordinate is the estimate of imprecision or RE). The position of this operating point is interpreted relative to the lines that define areas of "unacceptable," "poor," "marginal," "good," "excellent," and "world class" (Six Sigma) performance. See the PDF files on Westgard Web for details. We'll discuss the Method Decision Chart in detail in chapter 16.

References

1. Westgard JO, Hunt MR. Use and interpretation of common statistical tests in method comparison studies. Clin Chem 1973;19:49-57. See below for PDF files.

2. Westgard JO, Carey RN, Wold S. Criteria for judging precision and accuracy in method development and evaluation. Clin Chem 1974;20:825-33.

3. Westgard JO. A method evaluation decision chart (MEDx Chart) for judging method performance. Clin Lab Science. 1995;8:277-83.

4. Stockl D, Dewitte K, Thienpont M. Validity of linear regression in method comparison studies: limited by the statistical model or the quality of the analytical data? Clin Chem 1998;44:2340-6.

5. Cornbleet PJ, Gochman N. Incorrect least-squares regression coefficients in method-comparison analysis. Clin Chem 1979;25:432-8.

6. Bland JM, Altman DG. Statistical methods for assessing agreement beween two methods of clinical measurement. Lancet 1986;307-10.

7. Hyltoft-Petersen P, Stockl D, Blaabjerg O, Pedersen B, Birkemose E, Thienpont L, Flensted Lassen J, Kjeldsen J. Graphical interpretration of analytical data from comparison of a field method with a reference method by use of difference plots [opinion]. Clin Chem 1997;43:2039-46.

Online References:

The Method Validation data analysis tool kit
   http://www.westgard.com/mvtools.html

**Use and interpretation of common statistical tests in
method comparison studies.**
   http://www.westgard.com/method1.htm

Self-Assessment Questions:

○ Which calculations would you use for the data from a replication experiment?

○ Which calculations would you use with the data from a comparison of methods experiment?

○ What graphical presentations are associated with different types of data analysis?

○ What are the mean, SD, and CV on the basis of the following set of data[203, 202, 204, 201, 197, 200, 198, 196, 206, 198, 196, 192, 205, 195, 207, 198, 201, 195, 202, 195]?

○ What are the regression slope and intercept and the average bias on the basis of the following set of data [given as pairs where test result is 1st or y-value, comparison result is 2nd or x-value; 218,217; 161,161; 240,244; 193,193; 290,295; 117,118; 118,122; 203,204; 74,74; 114,116; 245,238; 262,260; 203,203; 218,207; 311,304; 362,353; 332,327; 428,423; 163,155; 268,257]?

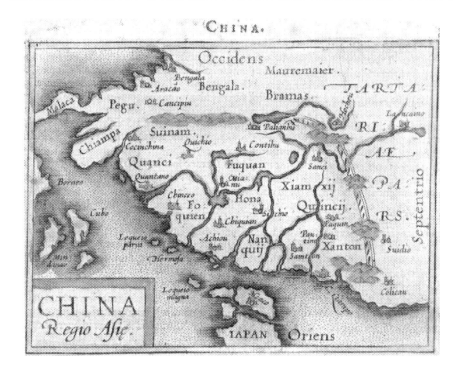

Another issue of perspective!
***CHINA**, by Philip Galle, Antwerp, 1595.*

China looks different in this map because North is to the right, not at the top. However, the Great Wall is still clearly shown. Your view of statistics is critical for their proper use and application. If you can remember that statistics are tools to estimate the *size* of analytical errors, then the important information will become clear.

8: How are the statistics calculated?

This chapter provides the equations that were so carefully avoided in the earlier chapter on data analysis tools. It is critical that you understand tests of statistical significance and their shortcomings in making judgments about method acceptability and performance claim verification. It's also important to understand the use and application of statistics found in general purpose statistical programs. You need to access the right calculations from those programs and sometimes it's necessary to look at the equations to confirm you're getting the right calculations.

Objectives:

○ Learn the statistical terms that are commonly found in method validation reports and manufacturer's claims for method performance.

○ Review the equations used to calculate those statistics.

○ Recognize critical aspects of the calculation and interpretation of the t and F-tests of significance and their capabilities for verifying a manufacturer's claims for method performance.

○ Identify the statistics commonly included in regression analysis, including the slope, y-intercept, standard error about the regression line, standard deviation of the slope, standard deviation of the intercept, and the correlation coefficient.

Lesson materials:

○ **MV – The Statistical Calculations**,
by James O. Westgard, PhD

Things to do:

○ Study the lesson.
○ Identify a computer program available for your routine work.
○ Find all the statistics in your computer program.

Method Validation: The Statistical Calculations

James O. Westgard, PhD

Statistics provide a tool by which many individual experimental results can be combined and summarized with a few numbers. This should be a great aid in clarifying the meaning of the experimental results. Yet, statistics often have the opposite effect, causing confusion rather than clarification. This usually occurs when the purpose of the statistical analysis is not well understood. In method validation, the objective should be to estimate the analytical errors from the results of the validation experiments. The statistics should provide information about the type and magnitude of analytical errors: otherwise they are of little value in interpreting the results of the validation study and in judging the acceptability of the method's performance.

A *statistic* is simply a number. It's a number that describes a series of *other* numbers from which it has been calculated. The mean ($\bar{x}$) of a set of numbers is calculated in the replication, recovery, and interference experiments. The standard deviation (**s**) is calculated in the replication experiment. These statistics are calculated from a limited number of observations, which are a subset or *statistical sample* of the population of interest. They provide estimates which are used to infer something about the *population* as a whole; yet these estimates are not necessarily identical with the numbers or *parameters* which describe the population. For example, $\bar{x}$ and s are statistics which are used to infer values to the parameters μ, the true mean, and σ, the true standard deviation. However, $\bar{x}$ and s may not be the same as μ and σ, especially when the number of measurements is small. Reliable inferences and conclusions can be made only when the experimental work is adequate and the statistical analysis and interpretation is properly done.

The proper use and interpretation of statistics is essential if the validation experiments are to enable objective decisions about the method performance. The statistics commonly used in method validation include mean, standard deviation, coefficient of variation, standard error of the mean, paired t-test, F-test, linear regression analysis, and correlation coefficient.

Mean, Standard Deviation, Coefficient of Variation

The *mean* ($\bar{x}$) is a measure of central tendency or location of a set of values. The *standard deviation* (s) is a measure of *dispersion* or spread of a set of measurements about the mean. The *coefficient of variation* (CV) expresses the standard deviation as a percentage of the mean. The equations are as follows:

$$\bar{x} = \frac{\Sigma x_i}{N}$$

$$s = \sqrt{\frac{\Sigma (x_i - \bar{x})^2}{N-1}}$$

$$CV = \frac{s\,(100\%)}{\bar{x}}$$

where x_i is an individual observation, $\bar{x}$ is the mean of the series of observations, and N is the total number of observations in the series.

The denominator of the second equation uses N-1 because this is an equation for the statistic s, rather than an equation for the parameter σ, in which case N would be used. The statistic s gives the best estimate of the parameter σ when N-1 is used and would underestimate σ if N were used. Of course, when N is large, it makes little difference whether N or N-1 is used.

N-1 also represents the number of *degrees of freedom* (df). This is a difficult concept. The degrees of freedom are defined as "the number of independent comparisons that can be made among N observations." This may also be thought of as the number of observations or measurements in a series minus the number of restrictions on the series. For example, if there were three measurements, only three simultaneous equations would be necessary to identify all three values. If the mean were calculated, then there would only be N-1 remaining independent equations, or N-1 independent comparisons, or N-1 degrees of freedom for a standard deviation. This becomes more obvious if N=1, in which case the single observation could be taken as an estimate of the mean, but it would not be possible to estimate a standard deviation. There is only one piece of information and it cannot be used to estimate two other quantities.

In using the standard deviation for describing a set of data, it is assumed that the *distribution* of the data fits a *Gaussian curve* or a *normal curve*. This is a symmetrical bell-shaped distribution which can be mathematically described by a specific equation in which the mean and the standard deviation are the variables. Statistics which assume a Gaussian distribution of a variable are called *parametric statistics*. Those that do not make any assumption about the nature of the distribution of a variable are called *nonparametric statistics*. All the statistics discussed here are parametric statistics.

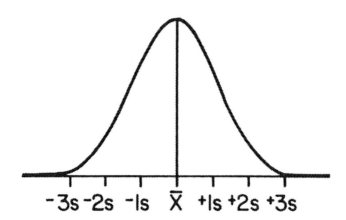

This figure shows a Gaussian curve. In a Gaussian curve, 68.2 percent of the observations will be within ± 1.0 s of the mean, 95.5 percent within ± 2.0 s of the mean, and 99.7 percent within ± 3.0 s of the mean. It is common to talk about a 95 percent *confidence interval* or *confidence range* and to estimate this by the mean ± 2.00 s, even though the exact multiplier should be 1.96 for a 95.0 percent interval.

Standard Error of the Mean

The dispersion of mean values is given by a statistic called the *standard error of the mean* (s_x), which is calculated from the equation:

$$s_x = \frac{s}{\sqrt{N}}$$

where s is the standard deviation representing the dispersion of single measurements as estimated from replicate measurements and N is the number of measurements included in the mean.

In validation experiments aimed at estimating systematic errors, such as the recovery and interference experiments, it is often useful to average the results from several measurements or samples. This reduces the effects of the random error of the method and permits an assessment of small systematic errors in a method which has a relatively large random error. The true mean of the measurements will be contained by a confidence interval around the experimental mean, as described by the following equation:

$$\mu = \overline{x} \pm t \frac{s}{\sqrt{N}}$$

The width of the interval is calculated from the standard error of the mean $(s/(N)^{1/2})$ and a multiplier (t). This multiplier must be appropriate for the degrees of freedom, which are N-1, and the desired confidence level, usually 90 percent, 95 percent, or 99 percent. The numerical value of the t multiplier is obtained from a statistics table, which usually lists t as a function of degrees of freedom and *probability* (p). The t-values for p=0.10 are used to calculate a 90 percent confidence interval, those for p=0.05 are used for a 95 percent confidence interval, and those for p=0.01 are used for a 99 percent confidence interval.

An example table of t-values is shown on page 91. Observe that the t-values for p=0.05 approach 1.96 as df approaches infinity. In general, a multiplier of 2 can be used to calculate a 95 percent confidence interval when df are 20 or more, and the interval will be correct to within four percent. This is the basis of the general usage of ± 2s as an estimate of the 95 percent confidence interval. Notice that as df gets smaller, especially below ten, t gets much larger. This is why it is important to obtain the correct t-value for experiments such as recovery and interference, where df or N-1 is likely to be small.

Here's an example of using the equation to calculate a confidence interval estimate of systematic error. Use the following data from a recovery experiment: 94 percent, 96 percent, 95 percent, 96 percent, 99 percent, 97 percent, 100 percent, 96 percent, and 98 percent. For these nine values, the mean recovery ($\overline{x}$) is 96.8 percent and the standard deviation (s) is 1.9 percent. Then the true mean recovery (μ) estimated with 95 percent confidence is

$$\mu = 96.8 \pm 2.31 \frac{1.9}{\sqrt{9}}$$

where 2.31 is the t-value for 8 df (N-1) and p=0.05, as obtained from the table on page 91. The interval from 95.3 percent to 98.3 percent has a 95 percent chance or probability of containing the true mean recovery. There is only a five percent chance or probability that the true mean recovery is outside this interval.

Similar calculations can be made for the interference experiment. For example, the following pairs of observations (baseline sample, test sample) show the effect of adding a suspected interference: 20, 23; 14, 20; 15, 20; 12, 15; 32, 35; 22, 26; 40, 42; 18, 23; and 16, 22. The interferences observed for the individual samples are 3, 6, 5, 3, 3, 4, 2, 5, and 6. The observed mean interference ($\overline{x}$) is 4.1 and the standard deviation (s) is 1.5. The true mean interference (μ) is estimated with 95 percent confidence as

$$\mu = 4.1 \pm 2.31 \frac{1.5}{\sqrt{9}}$$

where 2.31 is again the t-value for 8 df and p=0.05. The interval from 2.9 to 5.3 has a 95 percent chance of containing the true mean interference. There is only a five percent chance that the true mean interference is outside this interval.

The usefulness of stating a confidence interval as an estimate of systematic error should become apparent when comparing the results from the following two recovery experiments:

(A) $\bar{x}$ is 96.8 percent, the 95 percent confidence interval is 95.3 percent to 98.3 percent;

(B) $\bar{x}$ is 96.8 percent, the 95 percent confidence interval is 85.3 percent to 108.3 percent.

In experiment A, the data are sufficient to conclude that proportional systematic error exists because the confidence interval doesn't overlap the ideal value or 100 percent recovery. In experiment B, the data are not sufficient to support a conclusion that a proportional error exists because the confidence interval overlaps the ideal value of 100 percent.

Tests of Significance and Confidence Intervals

Statistical tests such as the t-test and the F-test are often used to determine whether a difference exists between two quantities which are estimates of performance parameters. These tests are called *tests of significance* and they test whether the experimental data are adequate to support a conclusion that a difference has been observed. The hypothesis being tested is called the *null hypothesis*, which states that there is no difference between the two quantities. When the test statistic (t or F) is large, the null hypothesis is disproved. The conclusion is that the difference is *statistically significant*. In practical terms, this means that a real difference has been observed. When the test statistic is small, the conclusion is that the null hypothesis stands and there is *no statistically significant difference* between the two quantities. No real difference has been observed.

Tests of significance provide similar information to that available from confidence intervals, and the similarity is useful in understanding them. When the calculated confidence interval for an estimate of a quantity does not overlap a specified value of interest, say zero, this means the estimate does not include that specified value and therefore is different from it. This is analogous to a test of significance which gives a large test statistic, thereby indicating a statistically significant difference. When the confidence overlaps the specified value of interest, this is analogous to the test of significance which indicates no statistically significant difference.

Paired t-test

A t-test can be used to test two means and determine whether a difference exists between them. There are both paired and unpaired forms of the t-test. This refers to whether the two means being compared come from the same statistical samples or from different statistical samples. For example, the paired t-test is used when there are pairs of measurements on one set of samples such as in the comparison of methods experiment in which every sample is analyzed by both the test and comparative method. The unpaired form is used when testing the difference between means in two separate sets of samples, such as the mean of the reference values for females versus the mean for males. Only the calculations of the paired form of the t-test are described here.

Three statistics are calculated. The *bias* is the difference between the two means:

$$\textbf{bias} = \bar{\textbf{y}} - \bar{\textbf{x}}$$

where the $\bar{y}$ and $\bar{x}$ are mean values. The *standard deviation of the differences* (SD_{diff}) is given by:

$$\textbf{SD}_{\textbf{diff}} = \sqrt{\frac{\Sigma[(\textbf{y}_i - \textbf{x}_i) - \textbf{bias}]^2}{\textbf{N} - 1}}$$

Finally, the *t-value* itself is calculated from the bias, SD_{diff}, and N using the equation:

$$\textbf{t} = \frac{\textbf{bias}}{\textbf{SD}_{\textbf{diff}} / \sqrt{\textbf{N}}}$$

This equation shows the nature of the t-value itself. It is a ratio of two terms, one that represents a systematic difference or error (bias) and another that represents a random error $(SD_{diff}/N^{1/2})$; in this case it has the form of a standard error of a mean because mean values are being tested). The value of t expresses the magnitude of the systematic error in multiples of random error. For example, a t-value of six would indicate that the systematic error term is six times larger than the random error term. This amount of systematic error is much larger than the amount that might be observable just due to the uncertainty

df	Two-sided intervals or tests		
	p=0.10	p=0.05	p=0.01
1	6.31	12.71	63.66
2	2.92	4.30	9.92
3	2.35	3.18	5.84
4	2.13	2.78	4.60
5	2.02	2.57	4.03
6	1.94	2.45	3.71
7	1.90	2.36	3.50
8	1.86	2.31	3.36
9	1.83	2.26	3.25
10	1.81	2.23	3.17
12	1.78	2.18	3.06
14	1.76	2.14	2.98
16	1.75	2.12	2.92
18	1.73	2.10	2.88
20	1.72	2.09	2.84
30	1.70	2.04	2.75
40	1.68	2.02	2.70
60	1.67	2.00	2.66
120	1.66	1.98	2.62
∞	1.64	1.96	2.58

t-table. Critical values of t for selected probabilities (p) and degrees of freedom (df).

in the experimental data. Ratios greater than two or three are not expected. If the ratio is that large, it is likely that the experimental data demonstrated a real difference between the mean values, or the presence of a systematic error.

A more exacting interpretation of the t-test is made by comparing the observed t-value from the first equation with a critical t-value which is obtained from a statistics table. The hypothesis being tested is that there is no difference between the two mean values (null hypothesis).

If the observed t-value is *greater* than the critical t-value found in the table, the null hypothesis is rejected, demonstrating that there is a difference between the two mean values, or that a systematic error has been observed. Usually, the statement made is that the difference or systematic error is statistically significant. This means that the difference observed is larger than that expected due to the uncertainty in the experimental data or the random error in the measurements. The conclusion is that the experimental data are sufficient to support a statement that a systematic error exists.

If the observed t-value is *less* than the critical t-value from the table, the null hypothesis is not rejected. There is no difference between the two mean values. The observed difference or systematic error is not statistically significant. This means that the experimental data does not support a conclusion that a systematic error exists.

The critical t-value is usually tabulated as a function of probability (p) and degrees of freedom (df). It is common to select a probability of 0.05 or 0.01 for test interpretation. For interpretation at p=0.05, there would be only a five percent chance or probability of 0.05 that the observed t-value would exceed the critical t-value due to the random errors in the measurements. This means that there is 95 percent confidence that the systematic error is real. For p=0.01, there would be only a one percent chance that the observation could occur due to random error, therefore there is 99 percent confidence that the systematic error is real. Degrees of freedom in the t-test are equal to N-1. For a comparison of methods experiment with 41 patient samples, there are 40 df. The critical t-value for p=0.05 and df=40 would be 2.02, as found in the table. For observed t-values greater than this, the experimental data demonstrate that a systematic error exists. For observed t-values less than this, the experimental data do not demonstrate the presence of a systematic error.

Note carefully that the interpretation says *nothing* about the acceptability of the method's performance, but only whether there is systematic error present. Acceptability will depend on the size of the systematic error, not the size of the t-value. There are situations where the t-value is large because the random error in the measurement is small or because the number of measurements is large. This is seen more easily when our previous equation is rearranged:

$$t = bias \frac{\sqrt{N}}{SD_{diff}}$$

If the bias is constant (and is not zero), t will get larger as N increases or as SD_{diff} decreases. On the other hand, when SD_{diff} is very large, or when N is very small, t will tend to be small. This causes difficulty in interpreting the t-value, a difficulty which is analogous to that in interpreting a blood pH value. Blood pH is a function of a ratio of bicarbonate and carbonic acid (or pCO_2). Information about these individual components is necessary for proper interpretation of the pH value. Similarly, information about the bias, SD_{diff}, and N must be given for the proper interpretation of the test.

Acceptability of performance should be judged based on the error estimates – bias and SD_{diff}. Ideal values for these statistics would be zero. The t-value could take on a wide range of values as bias and SD_{diff} approach their ideal values. Because of this, the t-value does not provide a reliable criterion for judging acceptability, though it is sometimes used in this manner. It is often erroneous to interpret a small t-value as an indicator of acceptable performance, or a large t-value as an indicator of unacceptable performance. **The only conclusion that should be drawn from the t-value is whether or not a systematic error has been shown to exist.**

F-Test

In method validation studies, the *F-test* is sometimes used to compare the variance of the test method with the variance of the comparative method. *Variance* is simply the square of the standard deviation. Whereas the t-test tells whether the difference between two mean values is statistically significant, the **F-test tells whether the difference in *variances* is statistically significant.** In short, the t-test is used for systematic error or inaccuracy, and the F-test is used for random error or imprecision.

To perform the F-test, the standard deviations of the test and comparative methods are squared and the larger variance is divided by the smaller variance, as shown below:

$$F = \frac{(s_1)^2}{(s_2)^2}$$

where s_1 is the larger s (or less precise method) and s_2 is the smaller s (or more precise method). The F-test is interpreted by comparing the calculated F-value with a critical F-value, which is obtained from a statistical table. The null hypothesis being tested is that there is no difference between the variances of the two methods. The null hypothesis is rejected when the observed F-value is greater than the critical F-value, and at that point, the difference in variances or random errors is said to be statistically significant.

The practical meaning is simply that the data are sufficient to show that the method in the numerator of the F-test equation has a larger random error than the method in the denominator. When the observed F-value is less than the critical F-value, the null hypothesis cannot be rejected. There is no difference between the variances or the random errors of the two methods.

For example, given a test method with s=5.0 (N=21) and a comparative method with s=4.0 (N=31), the calculated F-value is 1.56 (F=25/16). The accompanying table (*F-table*, following page) gives an abbrievated list of critical F-values for p=0.05. The column headings give the degrees of freedom in the numerator and the row headings give the degrees of freedom in the denominator. In both

F-table. Critical values of F for p=0.05 (probability) and selected degrees of freedom (df).

df for Denominator	5	10	15	20	30	60	∞
1	230.00	242.00	246.00	248.00	250.00	252.00	254.00
2	19.30	19.40	19.40	19.40	19.50	19.50	19.50
3	9.01	8.79	8.70	8.66	8.62	8.57	8.53
4	6.26	5.96	5.86	5.80	5.75	5.69	5.63
5	5.05	4.74	4.62	4.56	4.50	4.43	4.36
6	4.39	4.06	3.94	3.87	3.81	3.74	3.67
7	3.97	3.64	3.51	3.44	3.38	3.30	3.23
8	3.69	3.35	3.22	3.15	3.08	3.01	2.93
9	3.48	3.14	3.01	2.94	2.86	2.79	2.71
10	3.33	2.98	2.85	2.77	2.70	2.62	2.54
15	2.90	2.54	2.40	2.33	2.25	2.16	2.07
20	2.71	2.35	2.20	2.12	2.04	1.95	1.84
30	2.53	2.16	2.01	1.93	1.84	1.74	1.62
60	2.37	1.99	1.84	1.75	1.65	1.53	1.39
∞	2.21	1.83	1.67	1.57	1.46	1.32	1.00

cases, df equals N−1, where N is the number of measurements in the respective replication experiments. For the example here, the critical F-value is 1.93. The observed value is less than the critical value, meaning that there is no difference between the random errors of the two methods (at p=0.05).

Observe that the F-test interpretation says nothing about whether the random error of the test method is *acceptable*, but only whether it is different from that of the comparative method. The comparative method itself may or may not have acceptable random error, therefore testing the difference in random error between the test and comparative methods is really not relevant to the question of judging acceptability. Acceptability depends on the *size* of the random error, regardless of whether it is less than or greater than the random error of the comparative method.

Linear Regression Analysis

In the comparison of methods experiment, it is recommended that the data first be graphed, the test values on the y-axis and the comparative method values on the x-axis. A line can be drawn through the data points using visual judgment, and a qualitative assessment of the analytical errors can be made by visual inspection. This assessment can be made quantitatively by use of *linear regression analysis.*

This statistical procedure is sometimes referred to as least-squares analysis because of the technique used to determine the best location for the straight line through the set of data points. When this line is drawn manually, its location is judged by visually minimizing the distances of all points from the line. To find the best possible line, several could be drawn and the distances of all the points from each of the lines could be measured. The distances of the set of points from each line could then be totalled and the line with the lowest total should be the best line. In fact, the best line is that which minimizes the squares of the distances of the data points from the line, allowing the most distant points to have the greater effect on the line. This line is called the *least-squares line* and the statistical process is called *least-squares analysis*.

The straight line is described by the *regression equation*:

$$Y_1 = a + bx_1$$

where a is the y-intercept (the point where the line intersects the y-axis) and b is the slope (angle of the line on the graph).

The *slope* (b) is calculated from the equation:

$$b = \frac{N\Sigma x_i y_i - \Sigma x_i \Sigma y_i}{N\Sigma x_i^2 - (\Sigma x_i)^2}$$

Note that the term $(\Sigma x_i)^2$ means that the individual values are summed and the sum is then squared. This is not the same as Σx_i^2, which means that the individual values are squared first, then summed.

The *y-intercept* (a) is calculated from the equation:

$$a = \bar{y} - b\bar{x}$$

where $\bar{y}$ and $\bar{x}$ are the mean values for the patient samples by the test and comparative methods, respectively, and b is the slope from equation above.

The *standard deviation about the regression line* ($s_{y/x}$) is calculated from the equation:

$$s_{y/x} = \sqrt{\frac{\Sigma(y_i - Y_i)^2}{N - 2}}$$

This statistic is more commonly known as the *standard error* and sometimes as the *standard deviation of residuals*. It quantitates the scatter of the points about the regression line. To calculate $s_{y/x}$, the theoretical Y values corresponding to the x values are first calculated using the regression equation ($Y_i = a + bx_i$). The differences from the actual test values are calculated ($y_i - Y_i$), squared, and then summed. Observe that the standard deviation about the regression line equation listed directly above is very similar to the equation for calculating a standard deviation. There are two differences. The first is that Y_i is used in place of the mean value. This corresponds to taking the points on the regression line and calculating the differences or deviations of the actual points about the regression line. This is why we prefer to call the statistic the standard deviation *about the regression line*. The second difference from the standard deviation equation is the number of degrees of freedom in the denominator, which is N-2 here rather than N-1. This occurs because both the slope and intercept are calculated prior to calculating $s_{y/x}$, so there are two restrictions on the series of measurements, leaving N-2 remaining independent comparisons or degrees of freedom.

Two other statistics that are sometimes useful, though seldom seen in method validation reports in the literature, are the *standard deviation for the slope* (s_b) and the *standard deviation for the intercept* (s_a):

$$s_b = \frac{s_{y/x}}{\sqrt{\Sigma(x_i^2 - \bar{x})^2}}$$

$$s_a = s_{y/x} \sqrt{\frac{\Sigma x_i^2}{N\Sigma(x_i^2 - \bar{x})^2}}$$

These two statistics quantitate the spread of values for the slope and intercept, respectively, and permit calculation of confidence intervals for the slope and intercept.

Ideal values for the regression statistics would be 1.000 for the slope and zero for all the rest. These ideal values would be obtained only when the analytical results by the test method are exactly the same as those by the comparative method. Deviations of these statistics from their ideal values are therefore indications of analytical errors.

One of the most useful applications of the regression statistics is the calculation of systematic error. This can be done for any concentration in the range of concentrations studied in the comparison of methods experiment. For example, X_c may be a *medical decision level* where the interpretation of the test result is critical. The corresponding test method value, Y_c, could be calculated from the regression equation, substituting X_c for x_i and Y_c for y_i into the equation to give:

$$Y_c = a + b\,X_c$$

The systematic error (SE) is then given by the equation

$$SE = Y_c - X_c$$

when X_c equals $\bar{x}$, Y_c will equal $\bar{y}$, thus SE will equal the bias as estimated from the t-test. This suggests that regression analysis will provide the same estimate of systematic error, at least in the special case where an estimate is desired at the mean of the concentrations studied.

Correlation Coefficient

The *correlation coefficient* (r) can be calculated from the equation below, using the summation terms from the regression calculations:

$$r = \frac{N\Sigma x_i y_i - \Sigma x_i \Sigma y_i}{\sqrt{[N\Sigma x_i^2 - (\Sigma x_i)^2][N\Sigma y_i^2 - (\Sigma y_i)^2]}}$$

Values for r can vary from – 1.000 to + 1.000. A + 1.000 indicates perfect correlation, i.e. as x increases, y increases proportionally. A value of 0.000 indicates that there is no correlation, i.e. as x increases, y may increase or decrease. If r is – 1.000, perfect negative correlation exists. As x increases, y decreases proportionally. Situations of negative correlation will not be encountered in the comparison of methods experiment, which is the experiment where applications of r are usually seen.

Self-Assessment Questions

○ For a cholesterol method validation study, paired t-test analysis of the comparison of methods data gave the following results: bias= 1.74 mg/dL, SD_{diff}=5.90 mg/dL, N=81, and t=2.65. What is the critical t-value at p=0.05? Is the observed bias statistically significant? Is the observed bias clinically significant?

○ For a cholesterol method validation study, the test method has a standard deviation of 4.0 mg/dL and the comparison method had an SD of 5.0 mg/dL, both estimates based on 21 measurements on the same control material at a concentration approximately 200 mg/dL. What is the calculated F-value? What is the critical F-value? Is the observed difference in precision performance statistically significant? Is the observed difference clinically significant?

○ To verify a manufacturer's claim for precision, an F-test was calculated to compare the SD of 5.0 observed (N=31) in a replication experiment with the SD of 4.0 (N=31) claimed by the manufacturer. Have you verified the manufacturer's claim?

○ To verify a manufacturer's claim for precision, an F-test was calculated to compare the SD of 5.0 observed in the replication experiment (N=11) with the SD of 3.0 (N=11) claimed by the manufacturer? Have you verified the manufacturer's claim?

○ To verify a manufacturer's claim for accuracy, a t-test shows a bias of 1.5 mg/dL and t-value of 2.5 for a study of 40 patient samples compared to the same comparative method used by the manufacturer, who claimed there was no bias between the two methods. Have you verified the manufacturer's claim?

9: How is the reportable range of a method determined?

This chapter describes how reportable range can be determined using a series of standards with assigned values or using a series of dilutions of patient samples or patient pools. Graphical analysis of the data is recommended, along with visual assessment of the linear range. An online "linear-data plotter" can be used for either the standards with assigned values or the dilution series. Finally, the chapter provides a brief discussion of the experimental procedure for "calibration verification."

Objectives:

○ Learn a practical procedure for determining reportable range.

○ Identify important experimental factors.

○ Calculate and plot experimental data to determine reportable range.

○ Recognize the difference between reportable range and calibration verification.

Lesson materials:

○ **MV – The Linearity or Reportable Range experiment**

○ **Problem Set: Cholesterol method validation data**

○ **"Linear-data" plotter (www.westgard.com/mvtools.html)**

Things to do:

○ Study the materials.

○ Practice using the worksheets and online calculators.

○ Work the cholesterol problem set.

Method Validation:
The Linearity or Reportable Range Experiment

James O. Westgard, PhD and Elsa Quam, BS, MT(ASCP)

It is important to determine the reportable range of a laboratory method, i.e., the lowest and highest test results that are reliable and can be reported. Manufacturers make claims for reportable range by stating the lower and upper limits of the range. It is critical to check those claims, particularly when a method is assumed to be linear and "two-point calibration" is used.

Manufacturers provide directions and usually materials for calibrating their methods. Methods may require calibration with each analytical run, or only daily, weekly, monthly, or even longer intervals, or only when a new lot of reagents are put into use, depending on the manufacturer's documentation of method stability. Given long-term calibration, it may be necessary for the laboratory to periodically verify that calibration is correct, a function called "calibration verification" in the CLIA Final Rule.

Calibration is the procedure that determines the relationship between the signal generated by an analytical methodology and the test results that are reported. "Multi-point calibration" is required for methods that do not generate a linear response (e.g., immunoassay methods) and usually involves analyzing three to five (or even more) calibrator solutions and utilizing a curve-fitting routine to establish the calibration function.

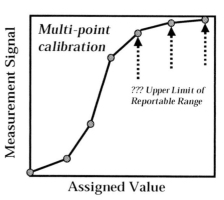

Some judgment may be required to assess the upper limit of the reportable range even when there are high calibrators in the upper range. The change in response may become so low in the upper range that the resolution of the measurement may no longer be satisfactory.

For example, are the changes between the test results meaningful between the two highest calibrators shown in the figure, or should the reportable range be restricted to the maximum value of the fifth calibrator?

In automated analyzers, "two-point calibration" is commonly used. Typically one calibrator provides a "zero-point" and the other a "set-point," as shown here. The assumption is that a linear calibration function can be drawn between the zero-point and the set-point and that the linear range extends beyond the set-point. How far beyond? The question should be answered by determining the reportable range.

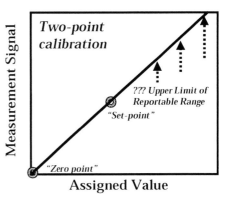

The experiment to be performed is often called a "linearity experiment," though there technically is no requirement that a method provide a linear response unless two-point calibration is being used. CLIA uses the term "reportable range" rather than "linear range," but it is common to also refer to this range as the "linear range," "analytical range," or "working range" for a method.

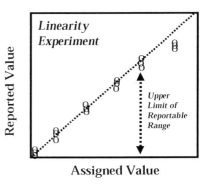

Because terminology varies in this area, it is important to understand the terms and meanings in the CLIA regulations.

Definitions of terms

The Final CLIA Rule [1] includes the following definitions (493.2) that are important in interpreting these requirements:

Calibration means a process of testing and adjusting an instrument or test system to establish a correlation between the measurement response and the concentration or amount of the substance that is being measured by the test procedure.

Calibration verification means the assaying of materials of known concentration in the same manner as patient samples to substantiate the instrument or test system's calibration throughout the reportable range for patient test results.

Note the relationship to the "reportable range," which is also defined in the Final CLIA Rule [1], as follows:

Reportable range means the span of test result values over which the laboratory can establish or verify the accuracy of the instrument or test system measurements response.

The College of American Pathologists makes use of different terms [2]:

Analytical measurement range (AMR) is the range of analyte values that a method can directly measure on the specimen without any dilution, concentration or other pretreatment not part of the usual assay process.

Clinically reportable range (CRR) is the range of analyte values that a method can measure, allowing for specimen dilution, concentration, or other pretreatment used to extend the direct analytical measurement range.

Recognize that AMR corresponds to the CLIA reportable range and the CRR provides additional practical information that can take into account the detection limit of a method and/or the extension of the AMR by verified procedures for diluting patient specimens. For example, the CRR low end for a method such as C-Reactive Protein (CRP) may be restricted to report values as less than 10 mg/L, rather than zero, to avoid confusion with results for a high sensitivity method (hs-CRP) where the values of interest are in the very low range, such as 1 to 5 mg/L. The high end of the CRR may allow dilution of patient specimens to extend the estimates of test values beyond the upper limit of the AMR, for example, for tests such as glucose and creatinine, where a dilution protocol may be in place to estimate values outside AMR.

Factors to consider

The linearity experiment involves a series of samples of known concentrations (assigned values) or a series of known dilutions of a highly elevated specimen or patient pool. The measured or reported test values are compared to the assigned values or to the dilution values, typically by plotting the measured values on the y-axis and the assigned or dilution values on the x-axis, as shown in the figure below.

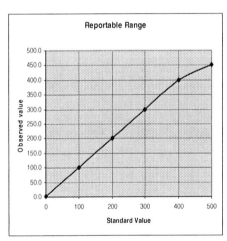
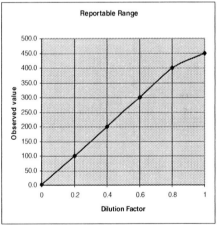

The reportable range is assessed by inspection of the linearity graph. That inspection may involve manually drawing the best straight line through the linear portion of the points, drawing a point-to-point line through all the points then comparing with the best straight line, or fitting a regression line through the points in the linear range. There are more complicated statistical calculations that are recommended in some guidelines, such as CLSI's EP-6 protocol [3] for evaluating the linearity of analytical methods. But it is commonly accepted that the reportable range can be adequately determined from a "visual" assessment, i.e., by manually drawing the best straight line that fits the lowest points in the series.

Number of levels

The Clinical Laboratory Standards Institute (CLSI) recommends a minimum of at least 4 – preferably 5 – different levels of concentrations [3]. More than 5 can be used, particularly if the upper limit of reportable range needs to be maximized, but we have found that 5 levels are convenient and almost always sufficient.

Materials

Standard solutions may be easy to prepare for some tests. For others, manufacturers and proficiency testing vendors may supply linearity sets having known values or known relationships between materials. Dilutions of patient specimens, or pools of patient specimens, may also be used and are often convenient and economical when high values are available. In some cases, e.g., TDMs, it may be necessary to spike a pool with the analyte to be measured in order to get the desired high level.

Diluent for use with patient specimens

Selection of the diluent is important when the matrix of the specimen needs to be maintained, e.g., when serum is the usual specimen type, it may be important to maintain a serum matrix for the series of diluted test samples. For general chemistry tests, water and saline will often be acceptable. For other tests, it may be better to use bovine or serum albumin preparations, specimens with low concentrations, or drug free serum. One way to decide on the diluent is to follow the manufacturer's recommendation for diluting out-of-range patient specimens.

Procedure for preparing dilutions

It is convenient to use two pools – one near the zero level or close to the detection limit and the other near or slightly above the expected upper limit of the reportable range. Determine the total volume needed for the analyses, select appropriate volumetric pipettes and then do the following:

1. Label the low pool "Pool 1" and the high pool "Pool 5."
2. Prepare Mixture 2 (75/25) with 3 parts Pool 1 + 1 part Pool 5.
3. Prepare Mixture 3 (50/50) with 2 parts Pool 1 + 2 parts Pool 5.
4. Prepare Mixture 4 (15/75) with 1 part Pool 1 + 3 parts Pool 5.

If more levels are desired, this dilution protocol can be modified, e.g., the two pools could be mixed 4 to 1, 3 to 2, 2 to 3, and 1 to 4 to give four intermediate levels for a total of six levels for the experiment.

Number of replicate measurements

CLSI recommends making 4 measurements on each specimen or pool. In practice, we have found that 3 replicates are generally sufficient, which means triplicates on the original high and low pools as well.

Data analysis

Plot the mean of the measured values on the y-axis versus the assigned values or relative values or dilution factors on the x-axis. First draw a line point-to-point through the entire analytical range. Then manually draw the best straight line through as many points as possible, making sure that the line adheres to the lower points or lower standards or dilution values. At concentrations where the straight line no longer adheres to the points, estimate the systematic error due to non-linearity. Compare that systematic error plus the expected random error at the concentration (2 SDs) to the allowable total error for the test.

Cholesterol example.

The data are as follows:

0 assigned, observed 0, 5, 10, average 5.0;
100 assigned, observed 95, 100, 105, average 100;
200 assigned, observed 200, 195, 205, average 200;
assigned 300, observed 310, 300, 290, average 300;
assigned 400, observed 380, 390, 400, average 390;
assigned 500, observed 470, 460, 480, average 470.

The accompanying figure shows the average values plotted on the y-axis against the assigned values on the x-axis.

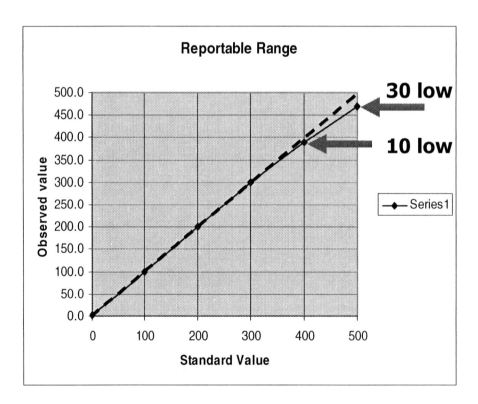

The solid line represents the line drawn point-to-point and the dashed line represents the straight line fitted to the points in the low to middle part of the range. Systematic differences are estimated to be 0 mg/dL at 300 mg/dL, 10 mg/dL at 400 mg/dL, and 30 mg/dL at 500 mg/dL. The reportable range clearly extends to 300 mg/dL, but does it extend to 400 mg/dL or 500 mg/dL?

- At 500 mg/dL, given a method with a CV of 3.0%, the SD would be 15 mg/dL and the 2SD estimate of random error would be 30 mg/dL. This means that a sample with a true value of 500 would, on average, be observed to be 470 mg/dL due to the systematic error from non-linearity. In addition, that value could be ±30 mg/dL due to random error, i.e., the expected value would be in the range from 440 to 500 mg/dL for a sample with a true value of 500 mg/dL. Given that the CLIA criterion for the allowable total error is 10%, which is 50 mg/dL at a level of 500 mg/dL, the errors that would be observed at 500 mg/dL could be larger than the allowable error, thus the reportable range should be restricted to a lower concentration.

- At 400 mg/dL, the SD would be 12 mg/dL, giving a 2SD estimate of random error as 24 mg/dL. A sample with a true value of 400 mg/dL would, on average, be observed to be 390 mg/dL due to the systematic error from non-linearity. Addition of the random error gives an expected range from 366 to 414 mg/dL, which means a result might be in error by as much as 34 mg/dL. The CLIA criterion of 10% provides an allowable total error of 40 mg/dL at 400 mg/dL, thus those expected results are correct with the allowable total error (34 mg/dL < 40 mg/dL), thus the reportable range does extend to 400 mg/dL.

Reportable Range and Calibration Verification

According to CLIA, calibration verification means the assaying of materials of known concentration in the same manner as patient samples to substantiate the instrument or test system's calibration throughout the reportable range for patient test results. For systems that are calibrated infrequently, calibration must be verified at least every 6 months and more often if there is a complete change of reagents, change of major parts or components, major maintenance, or an uncorrectable QC problem that demonstrates a shift of test results.

While the calibration verification experiment looks a lot like the experiment for reportable range, there is one important difference – the experiment must use materials with assigned values. Those materials may be a special calibration series from manufacturers or reagent vendors, calibrators that are run as unknowns like patient samples, control samples with assigned values, proficiency testing samples with known values, and even patient samples with assayed values [4]. The CLIA provision for assaying the materials like patient samples should not be considered a restriction on the experimental design. The use of replicate measurements will provide better information about possible systematic errors due to calibration.

The data analysis procedure should determine the differences between the observed and assigned values, then compare those differences with a criterion for acceptability, as defined by the laboratory. The approach can be similar to that outlined here for reportable range if replicate measurements were made and the mean of those values determined. If single measurements are made, then the observed differences can be compared directly to the allowable total error defined by CLIA.

References

1.   US Centers for Medicare & Medicaid Services (CMS). Medicare, Medicaid, and CLIA Programs: Laboratory Requirements Relating to quality Systems and Certain Personnel Qualifications. Final Rule. Fed Regist Jan 24 2003;16:3640-3714.

2.   CAP Laboratory Accreditation Checklists. http://www.cap.org

3.   CLSI EP6. Linearity of the Linearity of Quantitative Measurement Procedures: A Statistical Approach. Clinical Laboratory Standards Institute, Wayne PA, 2003.

4.   CMS State Operations Manual – Interpretative Guidelines: Appendix C. http://www.cms.hhs.gov/CLIA/ 03_Interpretive_Guidelines_for_Laboratories.asp

Self-Assessment Questions:

○ How many levels of materials are generally necessary for validating reportable range?

○ What's a practical way of preparing this series of materials?

○ How many replicate determinations are usually performed?

○ How are the data analyzed to assess the reportable range?

○ How are the data analyzed to assess linearity?

Problem Set – Cholesterol Method Validation Data: Linearity (used to determine reportable range)

A series of standard solutions having bottle values of 50, 100, 150, 200, 250, 300, 350, and 400 mg/dL were measured in triplicate. Prepare a plot of the data: assess the reportable range of this method. (The answers appear on page 300.)

Bottle Value	Measured Values		
	Result 1	Result 2	Result 3
50	50	50	49
100	102	101	101
150	148	159	147
200	190	200	198
250	237	261	251
300	300	314	310
350	345	352	343
400	396	395	372

10: How is the imprecision of a method determined?

Once you know the analytical range for reporting patient results, it's important to determine the imprecision of the method at concentrations where patient test results will be critically interpreted. This chapter describes how to perform a replication experiment, the factors that are important in the experimental procedure, and calculations and graphical display that are appropriate for the data.

Objectives:

○ Learn a practical procedure for estimating the imprecision of a method.

○ Identify the important experimental factors.

○ Calculate experimental data to assess imprecision.

Lesson materials:

○ **MV – The replication experiment,**
by James O. Westgard, PhD

○ **Problem set: Cholesterol method validation data**

Things to do:

○ Study the materials.

○ Practice using the online calculator.

○ Work the cholesterol problem set.

Method Validation:
The Replication Experiment

James O. Westgard, PhD

A replication experiment is performed to estimate the imprecision or random error of the analytical method. Methods of measurements are almost always subject to some random variation. Recall our bathroom scale illustration of random and systematic errors in *The experimental plan*, as well as the graphical descriptions in *The inner, hidden, deeper, secret meaning*. Repeat measurements will usually reveal slightly different results, sometimes a little higher, sometimes a little lower. Determining the amount of random error is usually one of the first steps in a method validation study.

A replication experiment is typically performed by obtaining test results on 20 samples of the same material and then calculating the mean, standard deviation, and coefficient of variation. The purpose is to observe the variation expected in a test result under the normal operating conditions of the laboratory. Ideally, the test variation should be small, i.e., all the answers on the repeated measurements should be nearly the same.

The replication experiment estimates the random error caused by factors that vary in the operation of the method, such as the pipetting of samples, the reaction conditions that depend on timing, mixing, temperature, and heating, and even the measurement itself. In non-automated systems, variation in the techniques of individual analysts may be a large contributor to the observed variation of a test. With automated systems, the lack of uniformity and the instability of instrument and reaction conditions may still cause small variations that may again show up as positive and negative variations in the final test results. While the exact effect can't be predicted at any moment, the distribution of these effects over time can be predicted to describe how large the random error might be.

Factors to consider

The amount of random error that will be observed depends on the experimental design because certain variables may not show up unless the right conditions are chosen. For example, when an experiment is performed in a short period of time, say within an analytical run, the effects of long term variation due to day-to-day changes in operating conditions will not be observed. Room temperature may be constant in that short time period, whereas it might vary more over a day, on different days, and in different seasons. Important factors for designing the experiment are the time period of the experiment, the matrix of the samples to be tested, the number and concentration of materials to be tested, and the number of samples to be analyzed. While it is expected that the number of analysts who perform the test may also be a factor, this variable is generally controlled during method validation studies and only one or a few well-trained analysts are involved in these studies.

Time period of experiment

The length of time over which the experiment is conducted is critical for the interpretation of the data and the conclusion that may be drawn. When samples are analyzed within a single analytical run, the "within-run" random error observed will generally be low (and optimistic) because the results are affected only by those factors that vary in this short time period. This is the best performance possible by the method; if this performance is not acceptable, the method should be rejected or the causes of random error need to be identified and eliminated before any further testing is carried out.

An experiment conducted over the period of one day, i.e., "within-day," will usually show more variation than a back-to-back within-run experiment unless the method is highly automated and very stable. An experiment conducted over a period of twenty days is expected to provide an even more realistic estimate of the variation that will be seen in patient samples over time. This estimate may be referred to as the "day-to-day," "between-day," or "total" imprecision of the method. CLSI prefers the term "total imprecision" perhaps because it implies that the within-day and between-day components of variability are included [1].

Matrix of sample

The other materials present in a sample constitute its matrix. For example, the matrix of interest for a laboratory test may be whole blood, serum, urine, or spinal fluid. While it may be of interest to measure glucose in each of these types of specimens, it will be difficult to find a single method for all these types of specimens. In evaluating method performance, it is important to use test samples that have a matrix as close as possible to the real specimen type of interest.

Test samples are commonly available as standard solutions, control solutions, patient pools, and individual patient samples. All can be used in a replication experiment, but each has certain advantages as well as limitations.

Standard solutions are often readily available for common chemistry analytes and can be made up to the concentrations of interest. The matrix of standard solutions is usually simpler than that of the real patient samples, e.g., the standard may be aqueous and the patient sample may be serum with a high protein concentration. Thus, an estimate of random error on a standard solution may be optimistic and is likely to represent the best performance available. Still, if that best performance is not satisfactory, a decision can be made to reject the method.

Control solutions or *control materials* can be obtained from commercial sources in convenient form and size and with long term stability. The matrix may be very similar to that of the patient matrix, but there still may be special effects due to stabilizers, lyophilization and reconstitution, and special additives to enhance the levels of certain tests, such as enzymes and lipids. It may get more difficult in the future to obtain control materials made from actual patient materials because of the need to test and document freedom from infectious diseases. See *Basic QC Practices* for a more extensive discussion of control materials.

Pools of fresh patient samples can often be used for short term testing, particularly within-run and within-day replication studies. Duplicates of fresh patient samples can be analyzed daily over long periods of time, but these samples will still reflect only the within-run and within-day components of imprecision. The between-day component will not be observed unless the duplicates are performed on different days, in which case the stability of the fresh sample must be demonstrated for the time period between the duplicates.

Number of materials and concentrations to be tested

The number of materials to be tested should depend on the concentrations that are critical for the medical use of the test. Generally, two or three materials should be selected to have analyte concentrations that are at medically important decision levels. A medical decision level represents a concentration where the medical interpretation of the test result is critical.

For cholesterol, medical decision levels are at 200 mg/dL and 240 mg/dL according to the NCEP recommendations for interpreting the result of a cholesterol test [2]. Glucose is typically interpreted at several medical decision levels, such as 50 mg/dL for hypoglycemia, 120 mg/dL for a fasting sample, 160 mg/dL for a glucose tolerance test, and at higher elevations such as 300 mg/dL for monitoring diabetic patients. For guidelines for a wide variety of tests, see the recommendations for Medical Decision Levels provided by Dr. Bernard Statland [3].

Number of test samples

It is commonly accepted that a minimum of 20 samples should be measured in the time period of interest. A larger number of samples will give a better estimate of the random error, but cost and time considerations often dictate that the data are evaluated at the earliest time or minimum period, then additional data are collected if necessary.

Data calculations

Random error is described quantitatively by calculating the mean ($\overline{x}$), standard deviation (s), and coefficient of variation (CV) from the number, n, of individual measurements, Σx_i, using these equations:

$$\overline{x} = \frac{\Sigma x_i}{n}$$

$$s = \sqrt{\frac{\Sigma(x_i - \overline{x})^2}{n - 1}}$$

$$CV = \left(\frac{s}{\overline{x}}\right) 100$$

Calculation programs are available on calculators, spreadsheets, statistical programs, and specialized method validation software, as well as online calculators available at Westgard Web – http://www.westgard.com/mvtools.html. It is also useful to prepare a histogram of the results to visually display the expected random variation and demonstrate just how large it might get for an individual measurement.

For patient specimens analyzed in duplicate, the standard deviation is calculated from the differences, d, between duplicates, using the following equation, where n is the number of different patient specimens:

$$s_{dup} = \sqrt{\frac{\Sigma d^2}{2n}}$$

Criteria for acceptable performance

Although these data calculations are simple, the issue of whether the calculated standard deviation represents acceptable analytical performance is not so simple. The judgment on acceptability depends on what amount of analytical error is allowable without affecting or limiting the use and interpretation of a test result [4,5]. As a starting point for defining the amount of error that is allowable, we recommend using the CLIA criteria for acceptability. These are available in Appendix 1.

For short-term imprecision, the within-run standard deviation ($s_{w\text{-run}}$) or the within-day standard deviation ($s_{w\text{-day}}$) should be 1/4 or less of the defined allowable total error to be acceptable, i.e.

$$s_{w\text{-run}} \text{ or } s_{w\text{-day}} < 0.25 \text{ TE}_a$$

For long-term imprecision, the total standard deviation (s_{tot}) should be 1/3 or less of the defined TE, i.e.

$$s_{tot} < 0.33 \text{ TE}_a$$

Similar judgments on acceptability can be made using a Method Decision Chart [6], which is available in PDF and Excel format at Westgard Web, and will be discussed in chapter 16.

Verification of Manufacturer's Claim

CLIA does not strictly require that a laboratory determine the acceptability of performance. Rather, CLIA says that the laboratory should verify the manufacturer's claim for precision. This can be done with the F-test, as follows:

- Obtain the expected SD and number of measurements used in the replication experiment from the manufacturer's claims (usually included in the instrument documentation), e.g., SD 3 mg/dL based on 31 measurements.

- Obtain the SD and number of measurements from your replication experiment, e.g., SD 4 mg/dL based on 21 measurements.

- Calculate the F-value, larger SD squared divided by smaller SD squared, i.e., $(4)^2/(3)^2 = 16/9 = 1.78$.

Page 119

- Look up the critical F-value for 20 degrees of freedom (df=N-1) in the numerator and 30 df in the denominator in the F-table on page 95, where the value found should be 1.93.

- In this case, the calculated-F is less than the critical-F, which indicates there is no real difference between the SD observed in the laboratory and the SD claimed by the manufacturer.

- Conclusion – manufacturer's claim has been verified!

Recommended minimum studies

Select at least 2 different control materials that represent low and high medical decision concentrations for the test of interest. Analyze 20 samples of each material within a run or within a day to obtain an estimate of short-term imprecision. Calculate the mean, standard deviation, and coefficient of variation for each material. Determine whether short-term imprecision is acceptable before proceeding with any further testing.

Analyze 1 sample of each of the 2 materials on 20 different days to estimate long-term imprecision. Calculate the mean, standard deviation, and coefficient of variation for each material. Determine whether long-term imprecision is acceptable.

Future considerations

Somewhat more elaborate experimental designs may be employed to provide more extensive information about the short-term and long-term components of variation. These designs often make use of statistical calculations known as Analysis of Variance (ANOVA), as illustrated in the CLSI protocols for precision [1,7]. The EP5 protocol is intended for manufacturers, whereas the EP15 protocol is intended for laboratory users. EP15 specifies a minimum of 3 replicates per day for a period of 5 days, giving a total of 15 measurements. To estimate the total imprecision, the calculations provide a way to determine within-run and between-run components which are then combined to provide the total imprecision. The necessary calculations are outlined in a worksheet in an appendix of EP15, plus there is an example set of data that shows how to verify a manufacturer's claim. Given that EP15 allows verification of precision with only 5 days data, it is likely that this will become the default protocol in many laboratories. For that reason, EP15 is discussed in detail in Chapter 19.

References:

1. CLSI CP5-A. Evaluation of Precision Performance of Quantitative Measurement Methods. Clinical and Laboratory Standards Institute, Wayne, PA 2004.

2. National Cholesterol Education Program Laboratory Standardization Panel. Current status of blood cholesterol measurement in clinical laboratories in the United States. Clin Chem 1988;34:193-201.

3. Statland BE. Clinical Decision Levels for Laboratory Tests, 2nd ed. Oradell NJ;Medical Economics Books, 1987.

4. Westgard JO, Carey RN, Wold S. Criteria for judging precision and accuracy in method development and evaluation. Clin Chem 1974;20:825-833.

5. Westgard JO, Burnett RW. Precision requirements for cost-effective operation of analytical processes. Clin Chem 1990;36:1629-1632.

6. Westgard JO. A method evaluation decision chart (MEDx Chart) for judging method performance. Clin Lab Science 1995;8:277-283.

7. CLSI EP15-A2. User Verification of Performance for Precision and Trueness. Clinical Laboratory Standards Institute, Wayne, PA, 2006.

Self-Assessment Questions:

○ How many levels or materials are needed for a replication study?

○ What is the minimum number of measurements generally collected?

○ What time period should the final replication experiment cover?

○ How are the data analyzed to estimate imprecision?

Problem Set – Cholesterol Method Validation Data: Replication (used to estimate imprecision or random error)

Two different control materials were assayed once per day for a period of 20 days. **Calculate the mean, SD, and coefficient of variation (%CV) for each control material. Prepare a histogram for each control.** (Answers appear on p.300.)

Day	Control A	Control B
1	203	240
2	202	250
3	204	235
4	201	248
5	197	236
6	200	234
7	198	242
8	196	244
9	206	243
10	198	240
11	196	233
12	192	237
13	205	243
14	190	234
15	207	241
16	198	240
17	201	249
18	195	232
19	209	231
20	186	241

11: How is the inaccuracy or bias of a method determined?

This chapter describes how a "comparison of methods" experiment is performed and how the data should be analyzed, emphasizing both statistical calculations and graphical displays. Regression and t-test statistics are considered, along with comparison and difference plots.

Objectives:

- ○ Learn a practical procedure for estimating the inaccuracy or bias of a method.

- ○ Identify the important experimental factors.

- ○ Compare statistical analyses and graphical presentations that are appropriate with sets of data that cover narrow and wide analytical ranges.

Lesson materials:

- ○ **MV – The comparison of methods experiment,**
  by James O. Westgard, PhD

- ○ **Problem set: Cholesterol method validation data**

Things to do:

- ○ Study the materials.

- ○ Practice using the online calculator.

- ○ Work the cholesterol problem set.

Method Validation:
The Comparison of Methods Experiment

James O. Westgard, PhD

A comparison of methods experiment is performed to estimate inaccuracy or systematic error. Review *The experimental plan* to see how this experiment fits together with the others. You perform this experiment by analyzing patient samples by the new method (test method) and a comparative method, then estimate the systematic errors on the basis of the differences observed between the methods. The systematic differences at critical medical decision concentrations are the errors of interest. However, information about the constant or proportional nature of the systematic error is also useful and often available from appropriate statistical calculations. Both the experimental design and the statistical calculations are critical for obtaining reliable estimates of systematic errors.

Factors to Consider

Comparative method

The analytical method that is used for comparison must be carefully selected because the interpretation of the experimental results will depend on the assumption that can be made about the correctness of results from the comparative method. When possible, a "reference method" should be chosen for the comparative method. This term has a specific meaning that infers a high quality method whose results are known to be correct through comparative studies with an accurate "definitive method" and/or through traceability of standard reference materials. Any differences between a test method and a reference method are assigned to the test method, i.e., the errors are attributed to the test method because the correctness of the reference method is well documented.

The term "comparative method" is a more general term and does not imply that the correctness of the method has been documented. Most routine laboratory methods fall into this latter category. Any differences between a test method and a routine method must be carefully interpreted. If the differences are small, then the two methods have the same relative accuracy. If the differences are large and medically unacceptable, then it is necessary to identify *which* method is inaccurate. Recovery and interference experiments can be employed to provide this additional information.

Number of patient specimens

A minimum of 40 different patient specimens should be tested by the two methods [1]. These specimens should be selected to cover the entire reportable range of the method and should represent the spectrum of diseases expected in routine application of the method. The actual *number* of specimens tested is less important than the *quality* of those specimens. Twenty specimens that are carefully selected on the basis of their observed concentrations will probably provide better information than a hundred specimens that are randomly received by the laboratory. The quality of the experiment and the estimates of systematic errors will depend more on getting a wide range of test results than a large number of test results.

The main advantage of a large number is to identify individual patient samples whose results do not agree because of interferences in an individual sample matrix. This is often of interest when the new method makes use of a different chemical reaction or a difference principle of measurement. Large numbers of specimens – 100 to 200 – are recommended to assess whether the new method's specificity is similar to that of the comparative method.

Single vs duplicate measurements

Common practice is to analyze each specimen once by both the test and comparative methods. However, there are advantages to making duplicate measurements whenever possible. Ideally, these duplicates should be two different samples (or cups) that are analyzed in different runs, or at least in different order (rather than back-to-back replicates on the same cup of sample). The duplicates provide a check on the validity of the measurements by the individual methods and help identify problems arising from sample mix-ups, transposition errors, and other mistakes. One or two such mistakes can have a major impact on the conclusions drawn from the experiment. At the very least, such mistakes cause much consternation over whether or not discrepant results represent the performance of the method or whether they are "outliers" that should be removed from the data set. Duplicate analyses can demonstrate whether or not these observed discrepancies are repeatable.

If duplicates are not performed, then it is critical to inspect the comparison results at the time they are collected, identify those specimens where the differences are large, and repeat those analyses while the specimens are still available.

Time period

Several different analytical runs on different days should be included to minimize any systematic errors that might occur in a single run. A minimum of 5 days is recommended [1], but it may be preferable to extend the experiment for a longer period of time. Since the long-term replication study will probably extend for 20 days, the comparison study can cover a similar period of time and will require only 2 to 5 patient specimens per day.

Specimen stability

Specimens should generally be analyzed within two hours of each other by the test and comparative methods [1], unless the specimens are known to have shorter stability, e.g., ammonia, lactate. Stability may be improved for some tests by adding preservatives, separating the serum or plasma from the cells, refrigeration, or freezing. Specimen handling must be carefully defined and systematized prior to beginning the comparison of methods study. Otherwise, the differences observed may be due to variables in the handling of specimens, rather than the systematic analytical errors that are the purpose of the experiment.

Data analysis

Here's where the going gets tough! There's a lot of debate and discussion about the right way to analyze data from a comparison of methods experiment [2]. This has been going on for as long as I've been a clinical chemist and seems to be a chronic problem that flares up with each new generation of laboratory scientists. We studied the use and interpretation of statistics in method comparison studies over thirty years ago [3,4] and the lessons we learned still apply today. Our intention here is to provide brief guidelines – the actual statistics are covered in more detail in the next chapter.

Graph the data

The most fundamental data analysis technique is to graph the comparison results and visually inspect the data. Ideally, this should be done *at the time the data are collected* in order to identify discrepant results that will complicate the data analysis. Any patient specimens with discrepant results between the test and comparative methods should be re-analyzed to confirm that the differences are real and not mistakes in recording the values or mix-ups of specimens.

If the two methods are expected to show one-to-one agreement, this initial graph may be a "difference plot" that displays the difference between the test minus comparative results on the y-axis versus the comparative result on the x-axis, such as shown in the accompanying figure. These differences should scatter around the line of zero differences, half being

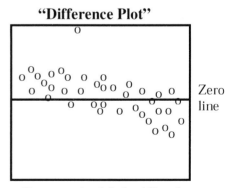

above and half being below. Any large differences will stand out and draw attention to those specimens whose results need to be confirmed by repeat measurements. Look for any outlying points that do not fall within the general pattern of the other data points. For example, there is one suspicious point in the difference plot. Note also that the points tend to scatter above the line at low concentrations and below the line at high concentrations, suggesting there may be some constant and/or proportional systematic errors present.

For methods that are not expected to show one-to-one agreement, for example enzyme analyses having different reaction conditions, the graph should be a "comparison plot" that displays the test result on the y-axis versus the comparison result on the x-axis, as shown by the second figure. As points are accumulated, a visual line of best fit should be drawn to show the general relationship between the methods and help identify discrepant results. Again, the purpose of this initial graphical inspection of data is to identify discrepant results in order to re-analyze specimens while they are fresh and still available. However, this type of graph is generally advantageous for showing the analytical range of data, the linearity of response over the range, and the general relationship between methods as shown by the angle of the line and its intercept with the y-axis.

"Comparison Plot"

Calculate appropriate statistics

While difference and comparison graphs provide visual impressions of the analytic errors between the test and comparative methods, numerical estimates of these errors can be obtained from statistical calculations. Remember *The inner, hidden, deeper, secret meaning* of method validation is error analysis. You need to know what kinds of errors are present and how large they might be. The statistical calculations will put more exact numbers on your visual impression of the errors.

Given that the purpose of the comparison of methods experiment is to assess inaccuracy, the statistics that are calculated should provide information about the systematic error at medically important decision concentrations. In addition, it would be useful to know the constant or proportional nature of that error (review *The experimental plan* for definitions of constant and proportional errors). This latter information is helpful in determining the cause or source of the systematic error and assessing the possibility of improving method performance. For additional discussion about the use and interpretation of statistics, see chapter 12 and the PDF files for reference 3.

For comparison results that cover a wide analytical range, e.g., glucose or cholesterol, linear regression statistics are preferred. These statistics allow estimation of the systematic error at more than one medical decision concentration to judge method acceptability and also provide information about the proportional or constant nature of the systematic error to assess possible sources of errors. Statistical programs typically provide linear regression or least-squares analysis calculations for the slope (b) and y-intercept (a) of the line of best fit and the standard deviation of the points about that line ($s_{y/x}$). The systematic error (SE) at a given medical decision concentration (X_c) is then determined by calculating the corresponding Y-value (Y_c) from the regression line, then taking the difference between Y_c and X_c, as follows:

$$Y_c = a + bX_c$$

$$SE = Y_c - X_c$$

For example, given a cholesterol comparison study where the regression line is $Y = 2.0 + 1.03X$, i.e., the y-intercept is 2.0 mg/dL and the slope is 1.03, the Y value corresponding to a critical decision level of 200 would be 208 ($Y = 2.0 + 1.03*200$), which means there is a systematic error of 8 mg/dL (208 – 200) at a critical decision level of 200 mg/dL.

It is also common to calculate the correlation coefficient, r, which is mainly useful for assessing whether the range of data is wide enough to provide good estimates of the slope and intercept, rather than judging the acceptability of the method [3]. When r is 0.99 or larger, simple linear regression calculations should provide reliable estimates of the slope and intercept. If r is smaller than 0.99, it would be better to collect additional data to expand the concentration range. Consider using t-test calculations to estimate the systematic error at the mean of the data, or utilize more complicated regression calculations that are appropriate for a narrower range of data [4].

For comparison results that cover a narrow analytical range, e.g., sodium or calcium, etc., it is usually best to calculate the average difference between results, which is the same as the difference between the averages by the two methods, also commonly called the bias. This calculated bias is typically available from statistical programs that provide paired t-test calculations. The calculations also include the standard deviation of the differences, which describes the distribution of these between-method differences, and a t-value (t), which can be used to interpret whether the data are sufficient to conclude that there really is a bias or difference between the methods. Chapters 8 and 12 discuss these statistics in detail.

For example, if the average of 40 analyses for sodium by the test method is 141.0 mmol/L and the average for the same specimens by the comparative method is 138.5, then the average systematic error, or bias, is 2.5 mmol/L (141.0 – 138.5). The algebraic sign of this bias is useful for showing which method is higher or lower, but it's the absolute value of the difference that is important for judging the acceptability of the method.

Criteria for acceptable performance

The judgment of acceptability depends on what amount of analytical error is allowable without affecting or limiting the use and interpretation of individual test results [5]. This is complicated by the fact that any individual test result is also subject to random error, thus the overall or total error (TE) is composed of systematic error (SE) plus random error (RE). This "total error" can be calculated as follows:

$$TE_{calc} = SE + RE$$

$$TE_{calc} = bias_{meas} + 3s_{meas}$$

where s_{meas} is the estimate of the method standard deviation from the replication experiment and $bias_{meas}$ is the average difference or difference between averages from t-test calculations or the difference between $Y_c - X_c$ where $Y_c = a + bX_c$ from regression statistics. Method performance is acceptable when this calculated total error (TE_{calc}) is less than the allowable total error (TE_a). Remember that the CLIA proficiency testing criteria for acceptable performance are in the form of allowable total errors and provide a good starting point for setting analytical quality requirements.

Similar judgments on acceptability can be made using the Method Decision Chart [6], which is described in chapter 16. This chart allows you to plot $bias_{meas}$ on the y-axis and s_{meas} on the x-axis, then judge acceptability by the location of this "operating point" relative to the lines for different total error criteria on the chart.

Verification of Manufacturer's Claim

CLIA does not strictly require that the laboratory judge the *acceptability* of any observed bias or systematic error relative to any quality standard, even to its own criteria for acceptable performance in proficiency testing. Instead, CLIA emphasizes the *verification of the manufacturer's claim* for accuracy (or inaccuracy, bias, systematic error). If a manufacturer claims there is no bias, t-test statistics will reveal whether or not the laboratory's data confirms the claim. If the calculated t-value from paired t-test statistics is less than the critical t-value, then no statistically significant or real bias has been observed. If a manufacturer claims a finite bias, then it is useful to determine the confidence interval for your estimate of bias and compare that with the manufacturer's claimed bias. If the manufacturer's claimed bias falls within the upper and lower confidence limits for the observed bias, then the claim is confirmed; if not, the claim has not been verified. Note one important simplification: if your observed bias is *less* than the manufacturer's claimed bias, you have verified the manufacturer's claim and no further statistical calculations are necessary.

For example, suppose a set of 41 patient comparisons for cholesterol gave a mean of 200 mg/dL, bias of 2.5 mg/dL, SD_{diff} of 4.3 mg/dL, and t-value of 2.58. If the manufacturer claims there is no bias, then apply the t-test to assess whether this is true. Look up the critical t-value for 40 degrees of freedom (N-1) and p=0.05 on page 91. Compare the calculated-t of 2.58 with the critical-t of 2.02 (df=40, p=0.05). Given calc-t > crit-t, you have observed a statistically significant, or real, bias. Your experimental results are different and do NOT verify the manufacturer's claim of zero bias.

Note, however, that the method might still perform acceptably since the actual bias of 2.5 mg/dL is small compared to CLIA's allowable total error of 10%.

If the manufacturer claimed a bias of 1.5 mg/dL, then it would be useful to calculate the confidence interval around your estimated bias of 2.5 mg/dL. The interval is calculated as follows: 2.5 mg/dL $\pm$ t$(SD_{diff})/N^{1/2}$, where the $\pm$ term is 2.02*4.3/6.4 or 1.4 mg/dL. Your estimate of bias is between 1.1 and 3.9 mg/dL, which includes the manufacturer's claimed bias of 1.5 mg/dL, therefore your experimental results have confirmed the manufacturer's claim.

Recommended minimum studies

Select 40 patient specimens to cover the full reportable range of the method. Analyze 8 specimens a day within 2 hours by the test and comparative methods. Graph the results immediately on a difference plot and inspect for discrepancies; reanalyze any specimens that give discrepant results to eliminate outliers and identify potential interferences. Continue the experiment for 5 days if no discrepant results are observed. Continue for another 5 days if discrepancies are observed during the first 5 days. Prepare a comparison plot of all the data to assess the range, outliers, and linearity. Calculate the correlation coefficient and if r is 0.99 or greater, calculate simple linear regression statistics and estimate the systematic error at medical decision concentrations. If r<0.975, estimate bias at the mean of the data from t-test statistics, or alternatively, from more sophisticated regression techniques [4]. Use the Method Decision Chart to combine the estimates of systematic and random error and make a judgment on the total error observed for the method.

Future Directions

The recommended number of patient samples for the comparison of methods experiment seems to lower by the year. CLIA's current guidance gives 20 as a "rule of thumb" for method validation experiments [7]. CLSI's EP15 guidance for user validation of "trueness" or bias also recommends a minimum of 20 patient samples. In addition, EP15 includes an alternate methodology that makes use of a minimum of 2 reference materials with assigned values that are to be measured in duplicate in 3 to 5 runs (see chapter 19). Reference materials here may include Certified Reference Materials, such as obtained from the US National Institute of Standards and Technology, but may also be proficiency testing samples, quality control materials, or peer-comparison materials having assigned values. Adoption of this alternate methodology using reference materials certainly lowers the bar and reduces the efforts needed to verify manufacturers' claims. You need to keep in mind that the real purpose of method validation is to make sure your laboratory is providing correct test results for the patients you serve, rather than just maintaining compliance with regulatory requirements. It is important to be thorough and make sure that your methods perform acceptably and provide the quality of testing required for patient care.

References:

1. CLSI EP9-A2. Method Comparison and Bias Estimation using Patient Samples. Clinical and Laboratory Standards Institute, Wayne, PA, 2002.

2. Hyltoft-Petersen P, Stockl D, Blaaberg O, Pedersen B, Birkemose E, Thienpont L, Flensted Lassen J, Kjeldsen J. Graphical interpretation of analytical data from a comparison of a field method with a reference method by use of difference plots. Clin Chem 1997;43:2039-2046.

3. Westgard JO, Hunt MR. Use and interpretation of common statistical tests in method-comparison studies. Clin Chem 1973;19:49-57.

4. Cornbleet PJ, Gochman N. Incorrect least-squares regression coefficients in method-comparison studies. Clin Chem 1979;25:432-438.

5. Westgard JO, Carey RN, Wold S. Criteria for judging precision and accuracy in method development and evaluation. Clin Chem 1974;20:825-833.

6. Westgard JO. A method evaluation decision chart (MEDx chart) for judging method performance. Clin Lab Science 1995;8:277-283.

7. CLIA Brochure: Validation of Performance Specifications. http://www.cms.hhs.gov/CLIA/05_CLIA_Brochures.asp

8. CLSI EP15-A2. User Verification of Performance for Precision and Trueness. Clinical and Laboratory Standards Institute, Wayne, PA, 2006.

Online References:

Method validation data analysis tool kit
> http://www.westgard.com/mvtools.html

Use and interpretation of common statistical tests in method-comparison studies.
> http://www.westgard.com/method1.htm

Self-Assessment Questions:

- What is the minimum number of specimens that are generally compared?

- How many replicate measurements are generally made?

- What time period should the experiment cover?

- How should the data be calculated when there are two medical decision levels?

- How should the data be plotted if there are two or more medical decision levels?

- What data calculations might be used if there is only a single decision level?

- How can data be plotted for only a single decision level?

Problem Set – Cholesterol Method Validation Data: Comparison of Methods

A comparison study was carried out using the Abell-Kendal method as the comparative method. Plot the comparison data, obtain the regression statistics, and determine the value of the correlation coefficient, r. (Answers on p.300.)

Sample	Abell-Kendal Comp. Method (X)	Test Method (Y)
1	217	203
2	224	213
3	298	279
4	172	160
5	198	189
6	274	262
7	253	238
8	197	275
9	226	211
10	151	149
11	166	151
12	163	151
13	215	205
14	151	133
15	263	252
16	226	212
17	239	226
18	162	147
19	253	235
20	159	157
21	261	250
22	247	231
23	261	238
24	184	179
25	295	284
26	250	232
27	201	196
28	209	212
29	286	275
30	158	142
31	288	281
32	161	145
33	183	171
34	252	239
35	285	277
36	194	190
37	240	230
38	180	177
39	297	275
40	210	188

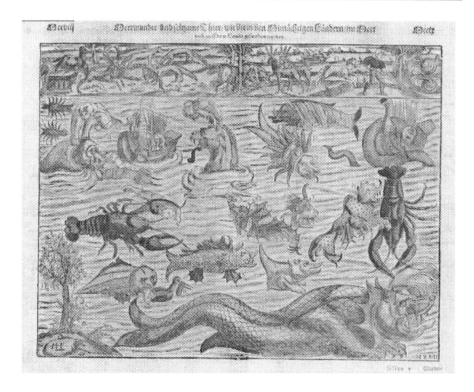

Munster's Monsters!
Sebastian Munster, 1598

We all have monsters to deal with, such as these ferocious sea creatures that decorated many maps in the 16ᵗʰ century. One of the modern monsters that we must face in the laboratory is called "statistics." Many fear statistics, but like Munster's Monsters, statistics are fanciful creatures that can be overcome by education and training. Learning to use statistics in method validation requires that you overcome your fears and adopt statistics as practical tools that help you summarize data and understand the meaning of all the numbers. The proper use of statistics is particularly important for understanding the results of the comparison of methods experiment.

12: How do you use statistics to estimate analytical errors?

This chapter provides more details about the analysis and interpretation of data from a comparison of methods experiment. It makes use of simulated data to demonstrate the behavior of statistical parameters in response to the different types of errors that may be observed in the data.

Objectives:

- Relate the statistics used to analyze the data from a comparison of methods experiment to the types of analytical errors occurring between the methods.

- Identify the limitations of t-test and regression statistics.

- Formulate a strategy to perform a proper analysis of data from a comparison of methods experiment.

Lesson materials:

- **MV – Statistical Sense, Sensitivity, and Significance,** by James O. Westgard, PhD

Things to do:

- Study the materials.
- Prepare a data set to demonstrate the effect of proportional error on t-test statistics and the difference plot.
- Prepare a data set to show the effect of a narrow range of data on regression statistics and the comparison plot.
- Examine a validation study published in the scientific literature and critique its use and application of statistics.

Method Validation:
Statistical Sense, Sensitivity, and Significance

James O. Westgard, PhD

Remember the 1ˢᵗ secret of method validation – it's all about error assessment. The 2ⁿᵈ secret is that statistics are just tools to estimate the size of those errors. The **data analysis toolkit** makes it easy for you to calculate the appropriate statistics and prepare corresponding graphics using online calculators and plotters. Even so, you still need to be careful in interpreting the statistics, particularly for data from the comparison of methods experiment.

Many years ago, we studied the use and interpretation of statistics for method-comparison data. We employed a data simulation approach to create data sets that had different types and magnitudes of analytical errors, then calculated regression statistics, t-test statistics, and the correlation coefficients for each of those data sets. We looked to see which statistics changed as the type and magnitude of analytical errors changed in the data sets.

Those results that were published in *Clinical Chemistry*[1] and the original paper is available on Westgard Web at **http://www.westgard.com/method1.htm**. In 2008, *Clinical Chemistry* recognized this paper as a "citation classic." [Clin Chem 2008:54;612] While that knowledge has been around for 30 years, it isn't being passed around in current education and training programs. Analysts still have great difficulty making sense of method comparison studies. The key to making statistics useful lies in understanding their sensitivity to different types of errors in the data. **Statistical sense relates to the sensitivity of statistics to errors.**

Simulation of errors in test results

Earlier glucose methods did not have the specificity of today's enzymatic methods. Because comparison studies between specific and non-specific glucose methods were appearing in the literature at that time, glucose was a good test for demonstrating how different types of analytical errors show up in the statistical results of method comparison studies.

We begin by constructing a data set of 41 specimens that would be typical for a hospital population, as shown in Table 1 by the reference method results in the 1st column. In a perfect world, the test method would give exactly the same results, as shown in the 2nd column. To demonstrate the effects of different types of errors, additional sets of comparison results can be created by manipulating the reference data set in specific ways.

- Random error can be simulated by alternately adding or subtracting 5 mg/dL to every data point in the reference set, as shown by the 3rd column of results. This is not truly random, at least not the normal or Gaussian random error expected for an analytical method, but it will suffice to demonstrate the effect. Additional data sets can be constructed for ± 2 mg/dL and ± 10 mg/dl to demonstrate the effect of changes in the size of the random error.

- Constant systematic error can be simulated by adding 10 mg/dL to every data point in the reference set, as shown by the 4th column. Additional data sets can be constructed by adding 2 mg/dL or 5 mg/dL to demonstrate the effect of changes in the size of the constant error.

- Proportional systematic error can be simulated by multiplying each result in the reference data set by 1.05. Additional data sets can be constructed using factors of 1.02 and 1.10 to demonstrate the effect of changes in size of the proportional error.

- Combinations of errors can be simulated by applying two or more of the above operations, as shown by the data in columns 6 through 8.

Table 1. Example simulated glucose data sets

Reference	Perfect	Random RE5	Constant CE5	Proportional PE5	RE & CE RE5+CE5	RE & PE RE5+PE5	RE & CE & PE RE5+CE5+PE5
40	40	35	45	38.00	45	33.25	42.75
60	60	65	65	57.00	65	61.75	61.75
80	80	75	85	76.00	85	71.25	80.75
90	90	95	95	85.50	95	90.25	90.25
100	100	95	105	95.00	105	90.25	99.75
110	110	115	115	104.50	115	109.25	109.25
120	120	115	125	114.00	125	109.25	118.75
125	125	130	130	118.75	130	123.50	123.50
130	130	125	135	123.50	135	118.75	128.25
135	135	140	140	128.25	140	133.00	133.00
140	140	135	145	133.00	145	128.25	137.75
145	145	150	150	137.75	150	142.50	142.50
150	150	145	155	142.50	155	137.75	147.25
155	155	160	160	147.25	160	152.00	152.00
165	165	160	170	156.75	170	152.00	161.50
170	170	175	175	161.50	175	166.25	166.25
175	175	170	180	166.25	180	161.50	171.00
180	180	185	185	171.00	185	175.75	175.75
185	185	180	190	175.75	190	171.00	180.50
190	190	195	195	180.50	195	185.25	185.25
195	195	190	200	185.25	200	180.50	190.00
200	200	205	205	190.00	205	194.75	194.75
205	205	200	210	194.75	210	190.00	199.50
210	210	215	215	199.50	215	204.25	204.25
215	215	210	220	204.25	220	199.50	209.00
220	220	225	225	209.00	225	213.75	213.75
225	225	220	230	213.75	230	209.00	218.50
230	230	235	235	218.50	235	223.25	223.25
235	235	230	240	223.25	240	218.50	228.00
240	240	245	245	228.00	245	232.75	232.75
245	245	240	250	232.75	250	228.00	237.50
250	250	255	255	237.50	255	242.25	242.25
260	260	255	265	247.00	265	242.25	251.75
270	270	275	275	256.50	275	261.25	261.25
280	280	275	285	266.00	285	261.25	270.75
290	290	295	295	275.50	295	280.25	280.25
300	300	295	305	285.00	305	280.25	289.75
320	320	325	325	304.00	325	308.75	308.75
340	340	335	345	323.00	345	318.25	327.75
380	380	385	385	361.00	385	365.75	365.75

Statistical analysis of the simulated data

These data sets are then subjected to the statistical calculations for regression (the slope, b; the y-intercept, a; and the standard deviation of the points about the regression line, $s_{y/x}$), paired t-test analysis (the average difference between methods, bias; the standard deviation of the differences, SD_{diff}; and the calculated t-value that is used to determine whether the bias is statistically significant or "real"), and finally the correlation coefficent, r.

Table 2. Effect of analytical errors on calculated results

Data set	RE	CE	PE	Slope	y-int	Sy/x	bias	SDdiff	t	r
1. Perfect	0	0	0	1.000	0.00	0.00	0.00	0.00	undefined	1.000
2. RE 2	2	0	0	1.001	-0.02	2.00	0.05	2.00	0.16	0.999
3. RE 5	5	0	0	1.001	-0.04	5.00	0.12	5.00	0.16	0.993
4. RE 10	10	0	0	1.003	-0.08	10.00	0.24	10.00	0.16	0.986
5. CE 2	0	2	0	1.000	2.00	0.00	2.00	0.00	undefined	1.000
6. CE 5	0	5	0	1.000	5.00	0.00	5.00	0.00	undefined	1.000
7. CE 10	0	10	0	1.000	10.00	0.00	10.00	0.00	undefined	1.000
8. PE 2	0	0	0	0.980	0.00	0.08	2.29	1.18	12.43	1.000
9. PE 5	0	0	5	0.950	0.00	0.08	5.72	2.95	12.42	1.000
10. PE 10	0	0	10	0.900	-0.04	0.14	11.45	5.88	12.47	1.000
11. RE5+CE2	5	2	0	1.001	1.96	5.00	2.12	5.00	2.72	0.996
12. RE5+CE5	5	5	0	1.002	4.92	5.02	5.10	5.03	6.50	0.996
13. RE5+CE10	5	10	0	1.002	9.95	5.02	10.10	5.03	12.86	0.996
14. RE10+CE2	10	2	0	1.003	1.92	10.00	2.24	10.00	1.44	0.986
15. RE10+CE5	10	5	0	1.003	4.92	10.00	5.24	10.00	3.36	0.986
16. RE10+CE10	10	10	0	1.003	9.92	10.00	10.24	10.00	6.56	0.986
17. RE2+PE5	2	0	5	0.951	-0.02	2.00	5.67	3.53	10.27	0.999
18. RE5+PE5	5	0	5	0.951	-0.04	5.00	5.59	5.76	6.27	0.996
19. RE10+PE5	10	0	5	0.953	-0.08	10.00	5.47	10.38	3.38	0.985
20. RE5+PE10	5	0	10	0.900	0.23	5.01	11.28	7.85	9.09	0.996
21. RE5+PE25	5	0	25	0.751	-0.02	5.00	28.45	15.58	11.62	0.994
22. RE5+PE50	5	0	50	0.501	-0.04	5.00	57.02	30.17	12.10	0.986
23. CE2+PE5	0	2	5	0.950	2.00	0.08	3.72	2.95	8.07	1.000
24. CE5+PE5	0	5	5	0.950	5.00	0.08	0.72	2.95	1.55	1.000
25. CE10+PE5	0	10	5	0.950	10.00	0.08	4.28	2.95	9.31	1.000
26. RE2+CE5+	2	5	10	0.905	4.99	2.03	6.37	6.28	6.50	0.999
27. RE10+CE2	10	2	5	0.953	1.89	10.01	3.48	10.5	12.12	0.984
28. RE5+CE10+PE2	5	10	2	0.981	9.96	4.99	7.84	5.18	9.69	0.996

The calculated statistics are shown in the 2ⁿᵈ table, where the leftmost column identifies the type and magnitude of the analytical errors in the data set (RE, random error; CE, constant error; PE, proportional error) and the next three columns show the magnitude of the errors. Each row provides the statistical results for the specific error condition or set of error conditions. Comparison of the error conditions and the statistical values allows us to match the type and magnitude of the errors to the estimates from the statistics.

No errors. Perfect comparison data would have exactly the same values for the test and reference methods. In a comparison plot, all the points would fall exactly on a line making a 45 degree angle and intersecting the axes at the origin. As shown in the table, the statistical results for this ideal situation show a value of 1.00 for the slope and correlation coefficient and values of 0.00 for all other statistics, except the t-value which is undefined (because it is a ratio of two terms that are both 0.00). *In a perfect world, the statistics have ideal values of 1.00 (slope, correlation coefficient) or 0.0 (y-intercept, $s_{y/x}$, bias, SD_{diff}). Deviations from those ideal values are indicators of errors.*

Random error. The effect of random error is shown in this figure for the data set where 5 mg/dL has been alternately added and subtracted from the reference set of values. Random error shows up in the plot as scatter in the points about the regression line. The statistical calculations in Table 2 show minimal changes in the slope, intercept, or bias, but the $s_{y/x}$ and SD_{diff} terms reflect directly the size of the random error. The correlation coefficent decreases as random error increases, but the changes in r are small and do not provide a direct estimate of random error in concentration units.

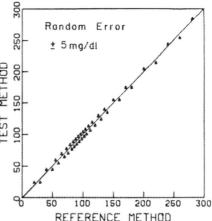

Constant error. The effect of constant error is shown in this next figure, where the regression line no longer goes through the origin. In this case, 10 mg/dL has been added to create a constant error and the magnitude of that error is correctly estimated by both the y-intercept from regression and the bias term from t-test analysis. Note that there is no change to the correlation coefficient.

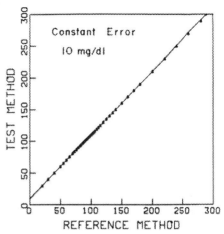

Proportional error. The effect of proportional error is shown for three situations where test results are lower than reference results by 2%, 5%, and 10%. Proportional error changes the steepness of the regression line and the exact magnitude of the error is estimated by the slope from regression analysis. Note that proportional error does not affect the y-intercept, $s_{y/x}$, and r, but does causes changes in both the bias and SD_{diff} terms in t-test analysis.

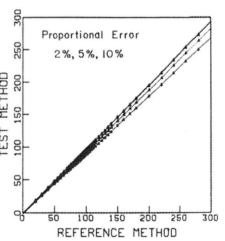

Sensitivity of statistics to types of errors

The behavior of these different statistics to the different types of errors is summarized in the table shown here. Random error is reflected by changes in $s_{y/x}$, SD_{diff}, and r. Constant error shows up in the y-intercept and the bias. Proportional error can be best estimated by the slope's deviation from ideal, but also causes changes in the bias and SD_{diff} from t-test analysis. That's a problem and the reason for the question mark in the table below. Proportional error confounds the interpretation of t-test statistics! There's also a problem with the correlation coefficient because it responds only to random error, not systematic errors, which are the errors of interest in the method comparison experiment. You can have an ideal correlation coefficient even if a method is inaccurate!

Sensitivity of Statistics	RE	CE	PE
Regression			
Slope, b	No	No	**Yes**
Y-intercept, a	No	**Yes**	No
SD about line, $s_{y/x}$	**Yes**	No	No
T-test			
Bias	No	**Yes**	*Yes?*
SDdiff	**Yes**	No	*Yes?*
Correlation coefficient			
r	*Yes?*	*No?*	*No?*

Estimation of random error. From the sensitivity table, it is apparent that there are three statistics that respond to random error. While this error was introduced into the test method by the data simulation, the statistics usually reflect the random error from both methods and sometimes even include additional scatter caused by differences in specificity between the two methods being compared. Therefore, the estimate of precision from the replication experiment is still important for characterizing the performance of an individual method.

Note that SD_{diff} is also influenced by proportional error, which means this statistic will not provide a specific estimate of random error. The other two statistics – $s_{y/x}$ and r – are sensitive only to random error, but they differ in their units and numerical values. It is most useful to estimate random error as a standard deviation and in concentration units as provided by $s_{y/x}$, rather than the unitless numbers provided by the correlation coefficient. A value of 5 mg/dL for $s_{y/x}$ can be readily interpreted in terms of the differences expected, for example, 95% of the differences will be within 2 times the value of $s_{y/x}$. A value of 0.996 for r does not provide an estimate of the size of random errors in a meaningful manner like a standard deviation term.

A further limitation of r is that it depends on the analytical range covered by the data. For example, in the two plots shown here, the random error is the same, ± 10 mg/dL, yet the values for r are very different, 0.986 vs 0.764. The plot on the left shows the wide range of data that would be expected from a hospital population, whereas the plot on the right shows the narrow range expected from a healthy population.

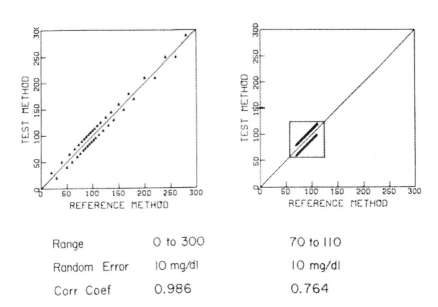

Range	0 to 300	70 to 110
Random Error	10 mg/dl	10 mg/dl
Corr Coef	0.986	0.764

The correlation coefficient is actually sensitive to the random error between methods (the scatter in the y direction) *relative to the range of analytical data in the x-direction.* A high correlation coefficient means that the y-scatter is small compared to the x-distribution. While this behavior makes the correlation coefficient useless for estimating analytical errors, it does provide a measure of reliability for the regression slope and intercept, i.e., a high r value means that the data cover a wide range relative to the scatter between methods, therefore the line through that data is well defined.

Estimation of constant error. The y-intercept from regression and the bias from t-test are the best statistics for estimating constant error. Both give the estimates in the units of concentration and provide similar values when proportional error is absent. However, proportional error does effect the bias term from t-test analysis, therefore that term does not provide a specific estimate of constant error. Instead it provides an overall estimate of systematic error that is reliable only at the mean of the data. Remember that bias is calculated as the difference between the mean of the test method results minus the mean of the comparative method results, which is the same as the average of the differences of all the individual specimens.

Estimation of proportional error. The slope from regression, as well as both the bias and SD_{diff} from t-test are all sensitive to proportional error. The fact that both the bias and SD_{diff} terms respond demonstrates these statistics cannot provide a specific estimate of proportional error. Both can be misleading because they also respond to other types of errors, i.e., the bias term responds to constant error and the SD_{diff} responds to random error. It would be best to avoid the use of t-test statistics when proportional error is present.

Regression provides the best estimate of proportional error. The difference between the slope and its ideal value of 1.00, expressed as a percentage, describes proportional error in the most useful way. For example, an observed slope of 0.95 indicates a proportional error of 5.0%.

Making Sense of Statistics

Correlation coefficient. The correlation coefficient provides information only about random error, even though the objective in a method comparison study is to estimate systematic error. Therefore, **the correlation coefficient is of little value for *estimating analytical errors* in a method-comparison experiment.** However, because r is sensitive to the range of data collected, **r is useful as a measure of the *reliability of the regression statistics*.** [Isn't it wonderful? A limitation can be turned into a useful feature once the behavior is properly understood.]

t-test statistics. The estimates of errors may be confounded by the presence of proportional error. There are two cases where the estimates of systematic error will be reliable: (1) if proportional error is absent, then the systematic error is constant throughout the concentration range; (2) if the mean of the patient results is close to the medical decision level of interest, then the overall estimate of constant and proportional error is reliable at the mean of the data, but that estimate of systematic error should not be extrapolated to other decision level concentrations.

- Inspection of a plot of test method values on the y-axis and comparison method values on the x-axis will usually reveal the presence of proportional error.

- If proportional error is NOT present, then the estimate of constant error should apply throughout the range of the data studied, but it would still be best to restrict the interpretation of decision levels near the mean of the data.

- If proportional error is present, it would be best to use regression statistics to estimate the systematic error at the decision levels of interest.

Regression statistics. It is ideal to have three statistical parameters that can each estimate a different type of error. Proportional error can be estimated from the slope, constant error by the y-intercept, and random error (between methods) from the standard deviation about the regression line. Systematic error can be estimated at any concentration using the regression equation, i.e., $Y_c = a + bX_c$, where X_c is the critical medical decision concentration and Y_c is the best estimate of that concentration by the test method. The difference between Y_c and X_c is the systematic error at that critical concentration, i.e., $Y_c - X_c = SE$.

The estimates of errors from regression statistics will not be reliable unless the data satisfies certain conditions and assumptions.

- Linearity is assumed, therefore you must inspect a plot of the comparison results to assure there is a linear relationship between the two methods. For example, the effect of non-linearity on the regression line is shown in the figure at right. Though it is obvious that there is some non-linearity at the high end, the calculations for linear regression will determine the best straight line through all the data. In this case, the points at the upper end will draw the line down, making the slope low and kicking up the y-intercept. The estimates of proportional error and constant error will both be corrupted by any non-linearity in the data.

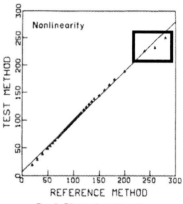

Fig. 5. Effect of nonlinearity

- Outliers can cause a similar problem! One or two points at the end of the line can exert undue influence by pulling the line towards those points and affecting both the slope and the y-intercept. The remedy again is to inspect a plot of the data to be sure there are no outliers.

- A narrow range of data is also a problem because a line cannot be well-defined by a cloud of data points. While this situation can sometimes be recognized from a plot of the data, the best alert is provided by the correlation coefficient. A low value for r, 0.99 or less in some references and 0.975 in others [2], indicates that the estimates of the slope and intercept may be affected by the scatter in the data. One remedy is to utilize more sophisticated regression techniques, such as Deming regression [3] or Passing-Bablock regression [4]. A simpler remedy is to utilize the bias estimate from t-test statistics and interpret the data at the mean of the patient results (assuming that the mean is close to the medical decision level of interest).

Statistical vs clinical significance. We have not included the t-value in the discussion so far because it does not provide an estimate of errors! This statistic is a "test of significance" that is mainly useful for deciding whether sufficient data have been collected to demonstrate that a difference exists. If the calculated t-value is greater than the critical t-value (which is 2.02 for the example data sets having 41 points), the observed bias is said to be statistically significant, which in practical terms means "real." If the calculated t-value is less than the critical t-value, then the data are not sufficient to demonstrate that a "statistically significance bias" exists between the test and reference sets of values.

From my perspective, this information on statistical significance is secondary in importance. The judgment on method acceptability must be made on clinical significance, not statistical significance. An error can be statistically significant, i.e., real, yet so small that it isn't clinically important. On the other hand, an error can be large and clinically important, yet the data may not be sufficient to demonstrate that it is statistically significant.

• Remember that the t-value is calculated as $t = bias * (N^{1/2} / SD_{diff})$, which shows that it is a ratio of systematic error (bias) divided by random error (SD_{diff}) multiplied by the square root of the number of paired samples ($N^{1/2}$). This is analogous to the equation for blood pH, where pH is a function of the ratio of bicarbonate to PCO_2 times a dissociation constant. A pH value by itself is difficult to interpret without having information about the bicarbonate and PCO_2 terms. Likewise, a t-value is difficult to make sense of unless you have information about the systematic and random error terms. Unfortunately, you will often find the t-value reported without any information being given about the bias or SD_{diff} terms.

- High t-values may result from bias being large, SD_{diff} being small, or N being large. A high t-value indicates that a real bias exists, however, that bias can be small and be statistically significant if SD_{diff} is small and/or N is large.

- Low t-values may result from bias being small, SD_{diff} being large, or N being small. A low t-value indicates that the data are not sufficient to demonstrate a real difference, therefore the conclusion is that no difference exists. However, a large bias may not be statistically significant if SD_{diff} is large and/ or N is small.

The acceptability of method performance depends on whether or not the errors will affect the clinical usefulness of the test results. Clinical significance depends on defining allowable limits of errors, then comparing the observed errors to those limits. If the observed errors are smaller than the allowable errors, method performance is acceptable. If the observed errors are larger than allowable, method performance is not acceptable.

What's the point?

You need to have a strategy for how to use statistics with data from the comparison of methods experiment if you expect to get good estimates of the analytical errors of interest! Here are the important parts of the data-analysis strategy:

- Plot the comparison data at the time of collection to identify any outliers while the patient samples are still available for further investigation. You can use either a difference plot (difference of test minus comparative results on y-axis vs. comparative results on x-axis) or the comparison graph (test method result as Y, comparative method result as X).

- Analyze the comparison data using regression statistics. Check the correlation coefficient (ideally should be 0.99 or greater) to be sure simple linear regression calculations provide reliable estimates of slope and intercept. Inspect the comparison graph to identify any problems with outliers and non-linearity. Estimate the systematic error at medically important decision levels (X_c) by calculating the corresponding Y_c values, then taking the differences (Y_c-X_c) as the estimate of the systematic errors at each medical decision level of interest.

- If regression statistics are not reliable, consider collecting more comparison results to extend the analytic range, then re-evaluate the correlation coefficent.

- Or, analyze the comparison data with t-test statistics. Restrict interpretation of results to a medical decision level near the mean of the data.

- Or, use more sophisticated regression calculations, such as Deming regression or Passing-Bablock regression, if specialized statistical programs are available.

Remember, statistical tests can provide estimates of errors upon which judgments can be made, but they are not a substitute for judgment. Clinical significance is determined by comparing the statistical estimates of errors to the defined allowable total error. A tool for doing this is the Method Decision Chart [5] that will be described in detail in chapter 16.

References

1. Westgard JO, Hunt MR. Use and interpretation of statistical tests in method-comparison studies. Clin Chem 1973;19:49-57.

2. Stockl D, Dewitte K, Thienpont M. Validity of linear regression in method comparison studies: Is it limited by the statistical model or the quality of the analytical input data? Clin Chem 1998;44:2340-6.

3. Cornbleet PJ, Gochman N. Incorrect least-squares regression coefficients in method-comparison analysis. Clin Chem 1979;25:432-8.

4. Passing H, Bablock W. A new biometrical procedure for testing the equality of measurements from two different analytical methods. J Clin Chem Clin Biochem 1983;21:709-720.

5. Westgard JO. A method evaluation decision chart (MEDx Chart) for judging method performance. Clin Lab Science 1995;8:277-83.

Self-Assessment Questions:

○ The following statistical summary was obtained for a glucose comparison of methods experiment:

$a = 5.23$ mg/dL, $b = 0.999$, $s_{y/x} = 7.23$ mg/dL, bias $= 5.13$ mg/dL, $SD_{diff} = 7.23$ mg/dL, $t = 8.03$, $r = 0.996$, $N = 128$.

- What is the proportional systematic error between methods?
- What is the constant systematic error between methods?
- What is the random error between methods?
- Why is there such good agreement between the estimates of error by regression and t-test statistics?
- Is the systematic error between methods statistically significant or "real"?
- What does the correlation coefficient tell you?

○ The following statistical summary was obtained for a urea nitrogen comparison of methods experiment:

$N = 316$, $a = -0.31$ mg/dL, $s_a = 0.23$ mg/dL, $b = 1.032$, $s_b = 0.009$, $s_{y/x} = 0.97$ mg/dL, $s_x = 13.2$ mg/dL, $r = 0.997$, bias $= 0.40$ mg/dL, $SD_{diff} = 1.08$ mg/dL, $t = 6.58$.

- What is the proportional systematic error between methods?
- What is the constant systematic error between methods?
- Why is it better to use the regression statistics to estimate errors rather than using t-test statistics?
- What is the 95% confidence interval for the y-intercept?
- Does the y-intercept differ significantly from the ideal value of 0.0?
- What is the 95% confidence interval for the slope?
- Does the slope differ significantly from the ideal value of 1.00?
- What does the correlation coefficient tell you?

13: How do you test for specific sources of inaccuracy?

This chapter describes experiments for interference and recovery, which are always needed if there is no comparative method available and often provide useful information in addition to the comparison of methods data. These experiments allow you to test specific sources that may be a cause of inaccuracy in the new method. Because these experiments are not required for unmodified non-waived methods, you may consider this chapter optional reading.

Objectives:

- ○ Learn practical procedures for validating interference and recovery.
- ○ Identify the important factors for performing interference and recovery studies.
- ○ Distinguish between interference and recovery experimental procedures.
- ○ Distinguish between the statistical calculations that are appropriate for data from interference and recovery experiments.
- ○ Describe constant error in the proper way.
- ○ Describe proportional error in the proper way

Lesson materials:

- ○ **MV – The interference and recovery experiments,** by James O. Westgard, PhD

- ○ **Problem set: Cholesterol method validation data**

Things to do:

- ○ Study the materials.
- ○ Work the cholesterol problem set.

Method Validation:
The Interference and Recovery Experiments

James O. Westgard, PhD

Method validation studies for unmodified moderate or high complexity tests tend to focus on the experiments for linearity or reportable range, replication, and comparison of methods, which have been described in previous chapters. However, our experimental plan recommends that interference and recovery experiments also be performed to estimate the effects of specific materials on the accuracy or systematic error of a method. These two experiments can be performed quickly to test for specific sources of errors. As such, they complement the estimates of error from the comparison of methods experiment. However, you may skip these materials, or parts of these materials, until those experiments become of interest to your applications.

Interference Experiment

Purpose

The interference experiment is performed to estimate the systematic error caused by other materials that may be present in the specimen being analyzed. We describe these errors as constant systematic errors because a given concentration of interfering material will generally cause a constant amount of error, regardless of the concentration of the sought-for analyte in the specimen being tested. As the concentration of interfering material changes, however, the size of the error is expected to change.

Factors to consider

The experimental procedure is illustrated in the figure at right. A pair of test samples are prepared for analysis by the method under study. The first test sample is prepared by adding a solution of the suspected interfering material (called "interferer," illustrated by "I" in the figure) to a patient specimen that contains the sought-for analyte (illustrated by "A" in the figure). A second test sample is prepared by

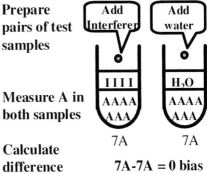

The Interference Experiment

diluting another aliquot of the same patient specimen with pure solvent or a diluting solution that doesn't contain the suspected interference. Both test samples are analyzed by the method of interest to see if there is any difference in values due to the addition of the suspected interference.

Analyte solution. Standard solutions, patient specimens, or patient pools can be used. We recommend a general procedure using patient specimens since they are conveniently available in a healthcare laboratory and contain the many substances found in the real specimen.

Replicates. It is good practice to make duplicate measurements on all samples because the systematic error is revealed by the differences between paired samples. Small differences may be obscured by the random error caused by the imprecision of the method. Making replicate measurements on the pairs of samples, or preparing pairs of samples for several specimens, permits the systematic error to be estimated from the differences in the average values, which will be less affected by the random error of the method.

Interferer solution. For soluble materials, it is convenient to use standard solutions to be able to introduce the interference at a known concentration. For some common interferences, such as lipemia and hemolysis, patient specimens or pools are often used.

Volume of interferer addition. The volume added should be small relative to the original test sample to minimize the dilution of the patient specimen. However, the *amount* of dilution is not as important as maintaining the *exact same* dilutions for the pair of test samples.

Pipetting performance. Precision is more important than accuracy because it is essential to maintain the same exact volumes in the pair of test samples.

Concentration of interferer material. The amount of interferer added should achieve a distinctly elevated level, preferably near the maximum concentration expected in the patient population. For example, in testing the ascorbic acid affects on a glucose method, a concentration near 15 mg/dL could be used because this represents the maximum expected concentration [1]. If an effect is observed at the maximum level, then it may also be of interest to test lower concentrations and determine the level at which the interference first invalidates the usefulness of the analytical results.

Interferences to be tested. The substances to be tested are selected from the manufacturer's performance claims, literature reports, summary articles on interfering materials, and data tabulations or databases, such as the extensive tabulation assembled by Young et al [2] which also contains a comprehensive bibliography.

It is also good practice to test common interferences such as bilirubin, hemolysis, lipemia, and the preservatives and anticoagulants used in specimen collection.

- Bilirubin can be tested by addition of a standard bilirubin solution.
- Hemolysis is often tested by removing one aliquot of a sample, then mechanically hemolyzing or freezing and thawing the specimen before removing a second aliquot.

- Lipemia can be tested by addition of a commercial fat emulsion or analyzing lipemia patient specimens before and after ultracentrifugation [3, see procedure recommended by CLSI].
- Additives to specimen collection tubes can be conveniently studied by drawing a whole blood specimen, then dispensing aliquots into a series of tubes containing the different additives.

Comparative method. We recommend that the interference samples also be analyzed by the comparative method, particularly when the comparative method is a routine service method. If both methods suffer from the same interference, this interference may not be sufficient grounds for rejecting the method. The test method may have other characteristics that would still improve the overall performance of the test. If the reason for changing methods is to get rid of an interference, then, of course, the interference data should be used to reject the new method.

Data calculations

The data analysis is equivalent to calculation of "paired t-test" statistics in a method comparison study and can be carried out with the same statistical program. However, the number of paired samples will be much smaller than the 40 specimens typically required in the comparison of methods study. Note also that regression statistics are not appropriate here because the data are not likely to demonstrate a wide analytical range. Here's a step-by-step procedure for calculating the data:

1. Tabulate the results for the pairs of samples.

   - Sample A: I added = 110, 112 mg/dL; dilution = 98, 102 mg/dL;
   - Sample B: I added = 106, 108 mg/dL; dilution = 93, 95 mg/dL;
   - Sample C: I added = 94, 98 mg/dL; dilution = 80, 84 mg/dL.

2. Calculate the average of the replicates.

   - Sample A: I added = 111 mg/dL; dilution = 100 mg/dL;
   - Sample B: I added = 107 mg/dL; dilution = 94 mg/dL;
   - Sample C: I added = 96 mg/dL; dilution = 82 mg/dL.

3. Calculate the differences between the results on the paired samples.

   - Sample A difference = 11 mg/dL;
   - Sample B difference = 13 mg/dL;
   - Sample C difference = 14 mg/dL.

4. Calculate the average difference for all the specimens tested at a given concentration or level of interference.

   - Average interference = 12.7 mg/dL.

Criterion for acceptable performance

The judgment on acceptability is made by comparing the observed systematic error with the amount of error that is allowable for the test. For example, a glucose test is supposed to be correct to within 10% according to the CLIA proficiency testing criteria for acceptable performance. At the upper end of the reference range (110 mg/dL), the allowable error would be 11.0 mg/dL. Because the observed interference of 12.7 mg/dL is greater than the allowable error, the performance of this method is not acceptable.

Recovery Experiment

Recovery studies are a classical technique for validating the performance of an analytical method. However, their use in clinical laboratories has been fraught with problems due to improper performance of the experiment, improper calculation of the data, and improper interpretation of the results. Recovery studies, therefore, are used selectively and do not have a high priority when another analytical method is available for comparison purposes. However, they may still be useful to help understand the nature of any bias revealed in the comparison of methods experiment. In the absence of a reliable comparison method, recovery studies should take on more importance.

Purpose

The recovery experiment is performed to estimate proportional systematic error. This is the type of error whose magnitude increases as the concentration of analyte increases. The error is often caused by a substance in the sample matrix that reacts with the sought-for analyte and therefore competes with the analytical reagent. The experiment may also be helpful for investigating calibration solutions whose assigned values are used to establish instrument set points.

Factors to consider

The experimental procedure is outlined in the accompanying figure. Note that pairs of test samples are prepared in a manner similar to the interference experiment. The important difference is that the solution added contains the sought-for analyte (shown as A) rather than an interfering material (shown as I in earlier figure). The solution added is often a standard or calibration solution of the sought-for analyte. Both test samples are then analyzed by the method of interest.

The Recovery Experiment

Volume of standard added. It is important to keep the volume of standard small relative to the volume of the original patient specimen to minimize the dilution of the original specimen matrix. Otherwise, the error may change as the matrix is diluted. We recommend that the dilution of the original specimen be no more than 10%. For a practical procedure, add 0.1 ml of standard solution to 0.9 ml or 1.0 ml of patient specimen.

Pipetting accuracy. This is critical because the concentration of analyte added will be calculated from the volume of standard and the volume of the original patient specimen. The experimental work must be carefully performed. High quality pipettes should be used and careful attention given to their cleaning, filling, and time for delivery.

Concentration of analyte added. One practical guideline is to add enough of the sought-for analyte to reach the next decision level for the test. For example, for glucose specimens with normal reference values in the range of 70 to 110 mg/dL, an addition of 50 mg/dL would raise the concentrations to 120 to 160 mg/dL, which are in the elevated range where medical interpretation of glucose tests will be critical. It is also important to consider the measurement variability of the method. A small level of addition will be more affected by the imprecision of the method than a large level of addition.

Concentration of standard solution. Given the importance of adding a small volume to minimize the effect of dilution, it will be desirable to use standard solutions with high concentrations. For our glucose example, a standard solution having 500 mg/dL would be needed to make an addition of 50 mg/dL, assuming 0.1 ml of standard is added to 0.9 ml of a patient specimen. A standard solution of 1,000 mg/dL would be needed to make an addition of 100 mg/dL. The concentration of the standard solution can be calculated once the volumes of the standard addition and the patient specimen are decided. If a general procedure of using 0.1 ml of standard and 0.9 ml of patient specimen is adopted, then the concentration of the standard solution will need to be 10 times the desired level of addition.

Number of replicate measurements per test specimen. Replicate measurements should be made on all test samples because the random error of the measurements often makes it difficult to observe small systematic errors. As a general rule, perform duplicate measurements. If the standard addition is low relative to the concentration of the original specimens, it may be desirable to perform triplicate or quadruplicate measurements.

Number of patient specimens tested. This depends on the competitive reaction that might cause a systematic error. For example, if the concern is to determine whether protein in a serum sample affects the analytical reaction, then only a few patient specimens need be investigated since they all contain protein. If the concern is to determine whether any drug metabolites affect recovery, then specimens from many different patients must be tested.

Verification of experimental technique. It is good practice to analyze the recovery samples by both the test and comparison methods. There are occasional problems caused by instability of the standard solutions, errors in preparation of samples, mixup of test samples, and mistakes in the data calculations. If the comparison method shows the same recovery as the test method, the results of this experiment are of limited value in assessing the acceptability of the test method.

Data calculations

Recovery should be expressed as a percentage because the experimental objective is to estimate proportional systematic error, which is a percentage type of error. Ideal recovery is 100.0%. The difference between 100 and the observed recovery (in percent) is the proportional systematic error. For example, a recovery of 95% corresponds to a proportional error of 5%.

Recovery calculations are tricky and often performed incorrectly, even in studies published in scientific journals. Here's a step-by-step procedure for calculating the data:

1. Calculate the amount of analyte added by multiplying the concentration of the standard solution by the dilution factor (ml standard)/(ml standard + ml specimen).

   - For example, for a calcium method, if 0.1 ml of a 20 mg/dL standard is added to 1.0 ml of serum, the amount added is 20*(0.1/1.1) or 1.82 mg/dL.

2. Average the results for the replicate measurements on each test sample.

   - Sample A addition = (11.4 +11.6)/2 = 11.5 mg/dL;
   - Sample A dilution = (9.7 + 9.9)/2 = 9.8 mg/dL;

- Sample B addition = (11.2 + 11.0)/2 = 11.1 mg/dL;
- Sample B dilution = (9.5 + 9.5)/2 = 9.5 mg/dL.

3. Take the difference between the sample with addition and the sample with dilution.

- Sample A addition = 11.5, Sample A dilution = 9.8, difference = 1.7 mg/dL;
- Sample B addition = 11.1, Sample B dilution = 9.5, difference = 1.6 mg/dL.

4. Calculate the recovery for each specimen as the "difference" [step 3] divided by the amount added [step 1].

- (1.7 mg/dL/1.82 mg/dL)100 = 93.4% recovery;
- (1.6 mg/dL/1.82 mg/dL)100 = 87.9% recovery;
[Note the variability of these estimates, which is probably due to method imprecision; it may be desirable to perform more replicate measurements or prepare more test samples.]

5. Average the recoveries from all the specimens tested.

- (93.4 + 87.9)/2 = 90.6% average recovery.

6. Calculate the proportional error.

- 100 - 90.6 = 9.4% proportional error.

Criterion for acceptable performance

The observed error is compared to the amount of error allowable for the test. For calcium, for example, the CLIA criterion for acceptable performance is 1 mg/dL. At the middle of the reference range, about 10 mg/dL, the allowable total error is 10%. Given that the observed proportional error is 9.4%, the performance of our method just meets the CLIA criterion for acceptability.

Summary comments about interference and recovery

Interference and recovery experiments can be used to assess the systematic errors of a method. They complement the comparison of methods experiment by allowing quick initial estimates of specific errors – the interference experiment for constant systematic error and the recovery experiment for proportional systematic error. In the absence of a comparison method, they provide an alternative way of estimating systematic errors.

The experimental techniques are similar, but the material being added is different. A suspected interfering material is added in the interference experiment, whereas the sought-for analyte is added in the recovery experiment.

The data calculations are different. The bias between paired samples should be calculated for the interference data, in a manner similar to the calculation of t-test statistics in the comparison of methods experiment. The average recovery in percent should be calculated from the recovery experiment, being careful to divide the difference between paired samples by the amount added, not by the total after addition. The proportional systematic error is the difference between 100% and the observed % recovery.

Interference experiments are generally useful to test the effects of common sample conditions, such as high bilirubin, hemolysis, lipemia, and additives to specimen collection tubes. Results in the literature are generally reliable.

Recovery studies are performed less frequently and results in the literature are difficult to interpret due to the lack of a standard way of calculating the data. A great deal of care and attention is necessary when performing recovery studies and also when interpreting the results.

When making judgments on method performance, the observed errors should be compared to the defined allowable error. The bias estimate from an interference experiment can be compared directly to an analytical quality requirement expressed in concentration units. The average recovery needs to be converted to proportional error (100 – %Recovery) and then compared to an analytical quality requirement expressed in percent.

References

1. Katz SM, DiSalvio TV. Ascorbic acid effects on serum glucose values. JAMA 1973;224:628.

2. Young DS. Effects of preanalytical variables on clinical laboratory tests. Washington DC:AACC Press, 1993. Also available at Young's Effects Online: http://www.fxol.org/aaccweb/

3. CLSI Document EP7-A. Interference testing in clinical chemistry. Approved Guideline. CLSI, 940 West Valley Road, Wayne, PA, 2002.

Self-Assessment Questions:

○ What's the difference between a recovery and interference experiment?

○ What common interferences are usually studied?

○ What is the proper way to calculate recovery?

Problem Set – Cholesterol Method Validation Data:
Recovery (used to estimate proportional systematic error)

Six different patient specimens (#1-6) were used. Two test samples (baseline, spiked) were prepared for each specimen. Each test sample was assayed 4 times. Baseline samples were prepared by diluting 0.9 mL of each patient specimen with 0.1 mL saline. Spiked samples were prepared by mixing 0.9 mL of each patient specimen with 0.1 mL of a 500 mg/dL cholesterol standard.

Calculate the amount of cholesterol added to the spiked samples, the amount recovered for each sample, and the average recovery for all 6 specimens. Remember, recovery is expressed as %. (Answers on p.300.)

Patient Specimens	Baseline Sample 0.9 mL specimen + 0.1 mL saline				Spiked Sample 0.9 specimen + 0.1 Chol standard			
	Result 1	Result 2	Result 3	Result 4	Result 1	Result 2	Result 3	Result 4
1	149	151	153	146	204	196	208	194
2	180	186	178	187	224	222	228	240
3	201	204	196	206	255	243	257	258
4	180	204	184	188	235	246	233	248
5	160	157	166	159	206	207	210	208
6	187	182	191	201	235	242	246	246

Problem Set – Cholesterol Method Validation Data: Interference (used to estimate constant systematic error)

Six different patient specimens (#1-6) were used. Two test samples (baseline, spiked) were prepared for each specimen. Each test sample was assayed 4 times. Baseline samples were prepared by diluting 0.9 mL of each patient specimen with 0.1 mL saline. Spiked samples were prepared by mixing 0.9 mL of each patient specimen with 0.1 mL of a 100 mg/dL bilirubin standard.

Calculate the amount of interference (bias) for each sample and the average bias for all the samples. Remember, interference is units of measure (mg/dL). (Answers on p.300.)

Patient Specimens	Baseline Sample 0.9 mL specimen + 0.1 mL saline				Spiked Sample 0.9 mL specimen + 0.1 mL Bili standard			
	Result 1	Result 2	Result 3	Result 4	Result 1	Result 2	Result 3	Result 4
1	206	213	223	215	221	222	230	229
2	220	228	223	210	233	241	228	237
3	299	287	297	297	306	304	302	296
4	169	171	167	178	186	184	181	183
5	250	248	257	252	242	265	271	262
6	227	221	224	230	236	229	237	242

14: What is the lowest test value that is reliable?

The reportable range experiment is used to characterize how high a test value can be and still be reliable, i.e., within the reportable range. The low end is characterized as a test value of zero. With certain tests, such as drugs of abuse, TDMs, and some cardiac markers, it is necessary to determine more exactly the minimum value that can be measured, i.e., the detection limit of the method. That is accomplished by performing an experiment for detection limit.

Objectives:

○ Learn a practical procedure for determining the detection limit of a method.

○ Distinguish between the concepts of Limit of Blank (LoB), Limit of Detection (LoD), Functional Sensitivity (FS), and Limit of Quantitation (LoQ).

○ Distinguish between the experimental procedures for these different characteristics.

Lesson materials:

○ **MV – The detection limit experiment,**
by James O. Westgard, PhD

○ **Problem set: Cholesterol method validation data**

Things to do:

○ Study the materials.

○ Work the cholesterol problem set.

Method Validation:
The Detection Limit Experiment

James O. Westgard, PhD

Purpose

The detection limit experiment is intended to estimate the lowest concentration of an analyte that can be measured. This low concentration limit is obviously of interest in forensic drug testing, where the presence or absence of a drug may be the critical information from the test. Analytical performance at low concentrations is also important for tumor markers, such as prostate specific antigen (PSA), where the monitoring of patient values after treatment may be useful for assessing "biochemical relapse" [1].

US laboratory regulations require that detection limit (or analytical sensitivity) be established only for non-waived methods that have been modified by the laboratory and test systems not subject to FDA clearance, such as methods developed in-house. Good laboratory practice dictates that detection limit be verified, when relevant, e.g., all forensic and therapeutic drug tests; TSH and similar immunoassay tests; cardiac markers such as the troponins; PSA and other cancer markers. Detection limit is not important for tests such as glucose, cholesterol, enzymes, and other constituents where there is a "normal" or reference range that is relevant for interpretation of the test results.

Terminology in this area is a mess! In making claims, manufacturers often use a variety of terms, such as sensitivity, analytical sensitivity, minimum detection limit, lower limit of detection, limit of blank, biologic detection limit, limit of detection, functional sensitivity, and limit of quantitation [2-6]. The CLSI guideline EP17-A [7] recommends standardizing the terminology with use of the following three parameters:

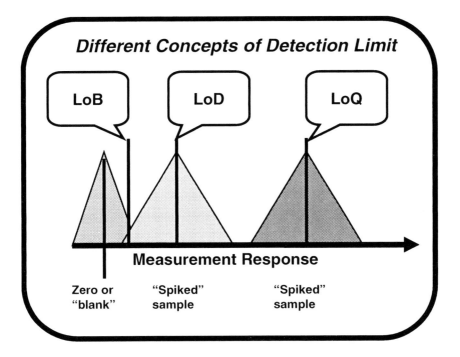

- **Limit of Blank (LoB)**: Highest measurement result that is likely to be observed (with a stated probability) for a blank sample; typically estimated as a 95% one-side confidence limit by the mean value of the blank plus 1.65 times the SD of the blank.

- **Limit of Detection (LoD)**: Lowest amount of analyte in a sample that can be detected with (stated) probability, although perhaps not quantified as an exact value; Estimated as a 95% one-sided confidence limit by the mean of the blank plus 1.65 time the SD of the blank plus 1.65 times the SD of a low concentration sample.

- **Limit of Quantification (LoQ) / Lower limit of quantification**: Lowest amount of analyte that can be quantitatively determined with stated acceptable precision and trueness, under stated experimental conditions; the analyte concentration at which the 95% limit of total error, i.e., bias plus 2*SD, meets the required or stated goal for allowable error.

Note that LoB replaces the earlier Lower Limit of Detection (LLD) term and is estimated in the same way. The main difference is that the multiplier for the SD is 1.65, rather than the 2 or 3 that was commonly used with LLD.

Likewise, LoD replaces the Biological Limit of Detection (BLD), with the main difference again being that the multiplier for the SD is 1.65, rather than the 2 or 3 commonly used with BLD.

LoQ is somewhat similar to the earlier Functional Sensitivity:

> *Functional Sensitivity (FS)*: The analyte concentration at which the method CV is 20%.[2]

Both represent analyte concentrations at which a certain level of analytical performance is achieved. For Functional Sensitivity, that level is the concentration at which a CV of 20% is achieved [2]. For LoQ, that level is the analyte concentration at which method bias plus 2 times the method SD satisfies a goal for allowable error. It is more complicated to estimate LoQ because it is more difficult to estimate method bias. It is also unlikely that many manufacturers will make a claim for LoQ because they are not required by the FDA to make labeling claims that define the quality that should be achieved by a test.

Factors to consider

A general description of the experimental procedure is provided in the accompanying figure. Two different kinds of samples are generally analyzed. One sample is a "blank" that has a zero concentration of the analyte of interest. The second is a "spiked" sample that has a low concentration of the analyte of interest. In some situations, particularly the estimation of FS and LoQ, several spiked samples may be needed at progressively higher analyte concentrations. Both the blank and spiked samples are measured repeatedly in a replication type of experiment, then the means and SDs are calculated from the values observed, and the estimate of detection limit is calculated from those results.

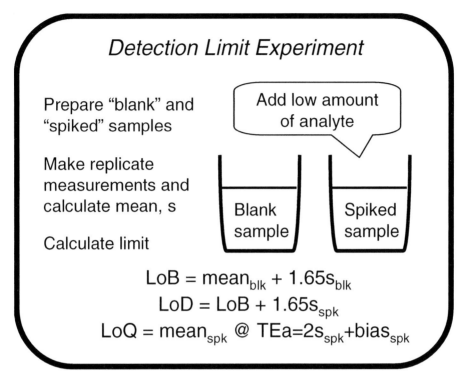

Blank solution. One aliquot of the blank solution is typically used for the "blank" and another aliquot is used to prepare a spiked sample. Ideally, the blank solution should have the same matrix as the regular patient samples. However, it is also common to use the "zero standard" from a series of calibrators as the blank and the lowest standard as the "spiked" sample.

Spiked sample. In verifying a claim for the detection limit of a method, the amount of analyte added to the blank solution should represent the detection concentration claimed by the manufacturer. To establish detection limit, it may be necessary to prepare several spiked samples whose concentrations are in the analytical range of the expected detection limit. For some tests, it may be of interest to use samples from patients who are free of disease following treatment (i.e., PSA sera from patients treated for prostate cancer)[4].

Number of replicate measurements. There is no hard and fast guideline, but 20 replicate measurements are often recommended in the literature. This number is reasonable given that the detection limit experiment is a special case of the replication experiment, where 20 measurements are generally accepted as the minimum. The CLSI guideline also suggests 20 replicates be made by a laboratory to verify a claim, but recommends a minimum of 60 by a manufacturer to establish a claim.

Time period of study. A within-run or short term study is often carried out when the main focus is the method performance on a blank solution. A longer time period, representing day-to-day performance, is recommended when the focus is on the "spiked" sample [2]. The CLSI guideline [7] recommends that LoD be estimated from data obtained over a period of "several days" and LoQ from data from at least 5 runs, assumed from over a 5 day period. Thus, multiple daily measurements should be made for a period of 5 days.

Quantity to be estimated. For laboratories, it will generally be most practical to verify or establish LoB or, preferably, LoD. In cases where the laboratory wants to verify claims for FS or LoQ, it will be best to follow the experimental protocol described in the manufacturer's claim or in the scientific study.

Example estimates

To illustrate the different concepts of detection limit (including FS), consider a case where 20 replicates provide an SD of 1.0 ug/L for a blank and also for low concentration spiked samples throughout the range from up to 10.0 ug/L. Assume this is a drug test, where the CLIA criterion for acceptable performance is 25%.

LoB will be equal to 1.65*1.0 ug/L or 1.65 ug/L.

LoD will be equal to LoB plus 1.65*1.0 ug/L, or 3.30 ug/L.

Functional Sensitivity will be equal to the concentration where the CV is 20%, which can be calculated from the equation for a CV, i.e., CV = 20% = SD*100/FS, where FS equals 1.0 ug/L*(100%/20%) or 5.0 ug/L.

For LoQ, assume that bias is 0.0, thus $TE_a = 25\% = 2*CV$ and a CV of 12.5% (25%/2) will be observed at a concentration of $SD*(100\%/12.5\%)$ or $1.0*8$ or 8.0 ug/L.

In practice, it is necessary to obtain experimental estimates of the SD for several sample concentrations, e.g., 0.0 ug/L, 3.0 ug/L, 6.0 ug/L and 9.0 ug/L. It is unlikely that the SDs will be exactly the same, so LoB will be estimated from the SD for the 0.0 ug/L sample, LoD using the additional SD from the 3.0 ug/L sample, FS from the 6.0 ug/L sample, and LoQ from the 9.0 ug/L sample. One approach for estimating FS and LoQ is to create a "precision profile," i.e., plot the CV vs concentration, draw a curve through the points, then interpolate that curve to identify the concentration corresponding to a CV of 20% (FS) and then the concentration where the CV is 12.5% (LoQ).

Verification of LoB and LoD claims

The CLSI guidelines recommend that laboratories verify claims by making 20 measurements. For LoB, the claim is verified if 3 or fewer of the 20 results on the blank sample exceed the claimed LoB. For LoD, the claim is verified if no more than 1 of the 20 results on a spiked sample (with the LoD concentration) is below the LoB. For a different number of replicate measurements, consult the CLSI guidelines [7].

Summary Comments

In validating a manufacturer's performance claim for detection limit, it is important to recognize the specific form of the claim, the data needed to verify that claim, and the data calculations appropriate for that claim. Many manufacturers choose LoB because it is the simplest to estimate and gives the lowest number – a marketing advantage. For medical applications, it is generally more useful to estimate LoD or LoQ. More manufacturers will make claims for LoD than LoQ, thus LoD is perhaps the most practical estimate. CLSI EP17-A provides the definitive guidelines for the concepts, experimental procedures, and data analysis, so most manufacturers will follow that guideline.

References

1. Diamandis EP, Yu J, Melegos DN. Ultrasensitive prostate-specific antigen assays and their clinical application. Clin Chem 1996;42:853-857.

2. Stamey TA. Lower limits of detection, biological detection limits, functional sensitivity, or residual cancer detection? Sensitivity reports on prostate-specific antigen assays mislead clinicians. Clin Chem 1996;42:849-852.

3. Lawson GM. Defining limit of detection and limit of quantitation as applied to drug of abuse testing: striving for a consensus. Clin Chem 1994;40:1218-1219.

4. Armbruster DA, Tillman MD, Hubbs LM. Limit of detection (LOD)/limit of quantitation (LOQ): Comparison of the empirical and the statistical methods exemplified with GC-MS assays of abused drugs. Clin Chem 1994;40:1233-1238.

5. Klee GG, Dodge LA, Zincke H., Oesterling JE. Measurement of serum prostate specific antigen using Imx prostate specific antigen assay. J Urol 1994;151:94-98.

6. Spencer CA, Takeuchi M, Kazarosyan M, MacKenzie F, Beckett GH, Wilkinson E. Interlaboratory/Intermethod differences in functional sensitivity of immunometric assays of thyrotropin (TSH) and impact on reliability of measurement of subnormal concentrations of TSH. Clin Chem 1995;41:367-374.

7. CLSI EP17-A. Protocols for Determination of Limits of Dection and Limits of Quantitation. Clniical Laboratory Standards Institue, Wayne PA, 2003.

Self-Assessment Questions:

○ When do you need to perform a detection limit experiment?

○ Which estimate of detection limit will generally give the highest value?

○ Why is the limit of detection (LoD) always higher than the limit of blank (LoB)?

Problem Set – Cholesterol Method Validation Data: Detection Limit

From the data below, calculate the limit of blank (LoB), limit of detection (LoD), and functional sensitivity (FS). (Answers can be found on page 300.)

Standard 0	Standard 2	Standard 4	Standard 6	Standard 8
-0.23	2.84	5.51	6.46	6.92
0.12	2.26	5.07	5.14	6.29
-0.40	1.25	3.15	3.78	8.67
0.13	3.52	2.72	7.28	7.86
0.05	1.95	3.67	6.20	5.24
0.18	2.71	5.35	5.00	7.38
-0.41	3.07	5.22	5.54	7.41
0.20	2.47	4.46	6.44	6.06
-0.32	1.95	2.55	6.71	7.53
-0.08	1.94	3.61	7.17	10.11
-0.41	1.93	3.79	4.92	8.70
-0.39	2.45	3.21	4.40	6.37
-0.32	2.38	3.42	6.11	7.54
-0.37	1.37	4.73	7.51	9.30
-0.17	1.58	4.07	6.38	8.10
0.38	2.46	3.47	5.55	7.87
-0.31	2.55	3.28	8.19	8.20
-0.41	2.57	5.67	8.48	7.99
0.10	2.27	4.99	5.45	9.38
-0.30	1.57	4.42	7.61	8.22

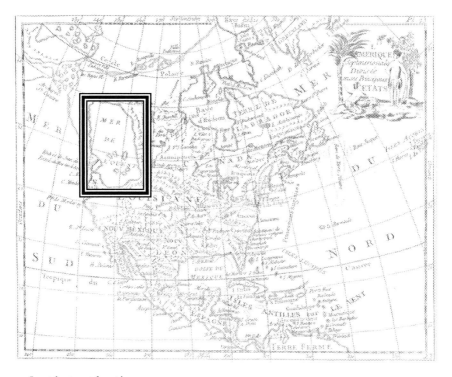

Last but not least!
L'AMERIQUE SEPTENTRIONALE, *by De la Porte, Paris, 1786.*

The Pacific Northwest was one of the last areas to be explored and gave rise to some of the biggest myths, such as the large "Sea of the West" shown on this map. The experiments on interference, recovery, and detection limit are likely to be the last experiments you explore, too. However, they are critical for certain methods in your laboratory. Remember that they're discussed in these last two chapters; come back and review this material when it becomes relevant for your own applications.

15: How is the reference interval of a method verified?

One last consideration is to verify that the reference interval is appropriate for the patient population. In this chapter, Patricia L. Barry, BS, MT(ASCP), presents a practical procedure for assessing the validity of the manufacturer's recommendations for reference intervals.

Objectives:

- ○ Describe 4 approaches for verifying or transferring reference intervals.
- ○ Identify the conditions for application of the different approaches.
- ○ Compare the data requirements of the different approaches.
- ○ Compare the data calculations and presentations.
- ○ Organize the approaches into a plan for practical application.

Lesson materials:

- ○ **MV – Reference interval transference**, by Patricia L. Barry, BS, MT(ASCP) and James O. Westgard, PhD

Things to do:

- ○ Study the materials.
- ○ Review a manufacturer's recommendations for reference intervals for a test of interest.
- ○ Assess which approach would be appropriate to verify or transfer the manufacturer's recommendation.

Method Validation:
Reference Interval Transference

Patricia L. Barry, BS, MT(ASCP), and James O. Westgard, PhD

Purpose

The reference interval is the last characteristic to be studied in the method validation process. It is generally studied last because the reference interval itself doesn't enter into the decision on method acceptability and the study isn't needed when method performance is unacceptable. If method performance is acceptable, then it is important to assess the reference interval(s) to support the interpretation of patient test results.

Background

A reference interval is typically established by assaying specimens that are obtained from individuals that meet carefully defined criteria (reference sample group). Protocols such as those of the International Federation of Clinical Chemistry (IFCC) Expert Panel on Theory of Reference Values [1-6] and the Clinical Laboratory Standards Institute (CLSI) [7] delineate comprehensive, systematic processes that use carefully selected reference sample groups to establish reference intervals. These protocols typically need a minimum of 120 reference individuals for each group (or subgroup) that needs to be characterized.

For example, to establish a reference interval for hemoglobin – a test that is gender dependent – the laboratory would need to obtain hemoglobin results on 240 reference individuals (120 men and 120 women). These individuals are typically recruited from the general regional population (essentially the facility's market-base) and then selected for inclusion in the study using carefully defined criteria. The selection is often accomplished by administering a health questionnaire. Sometimes a physical examination is also required as a way to determine acceptability for inclusion.

The establishment of reference intervals requires careful planning, control, and documentation of each aspect of the study. Thus, the resulting reference intervals are well-characterized in terms of the variation attributable to pre-analytical and analytical factors. These formal protocols are particularly helpful when a laboratory needs to establish its own reference interval for a particular test. This situation may occur if a laboratory has modified a previously FDA-approved method or developed an in-house test. Unfortunately, these protocols are resource-intensive and can be prohibitive for smaller facilities. Even large laboratories are finding it increasingly difficult to conduct these comprehensive studies cost-effectively. Therefore, laboratories are more and more reliant on manufacturers to establish scientifically sound reference intervals that can be verified using simpler, less labor-intensive, and lower cost approaches.

In this chapter, the focus is on the *transference* of reference intervals, which requires considerably less effort and less data than necessary for the *establishment* of reference intervals. The reference interval that is of most interest during the method validation process is one that describes the test values typically observed in a "healthy" population. This interval has historically been referred to as the "normal range" and is derived by assaying specimens from individuals who meet criteria for "good" health (e.g., "have no known health problems, are ambulatory, not on any regular medication regimen, have a weight within the recommended norms, etc."). The test results (reference values) from this sample group are analyzed statistically to determine an interval of values that includes a specified percentage of all the values (reference interval) from the sample group. By tradition, this interval includes 95% of the values (usually the central 95%). A pair of test values (called the lower and upper reference limits) represents the boundaries of the interval. Patient results falling outside the reference limits are typically flagged in some way as "abnormal" results.

Transference approaches to consider

The CLSI Approved Guideline C28-A2 [7] describes different ways for a laboratory to validate the "transference" of established reference intervals to the individual laboratory:

1. Divine judgment.

The acceptability of the transfer may be subjectively assessed on the basis of consistency between the "demographics and geographics" of the study population(s) and the demographics of the laboratory's test population(s). The laboratory simply reviews the information submitted and subjectively verifies that the reference intervals are applicable to the adopting laboratory's patient population and test methods. To do this, all the information about the original study should be requested and made available to the adopting laboratory. This includes the demographics of the reference sample group, the selection process, pre-analytical conditions of the study such as subject preparation and specimen collection and handling techniques, the analytical system used, and the statistical method used to establish the intervals. Sometimes it is useful to request the original reference values and to re-analyze them to verify the original statistical analysis. Most cases for transference involve adoption of intervals from another laboratory using the same analytical system or intervals established by the method manufacturer.

- CLIA Final Rule regulations permit the Medical Director of a laboratory to make this assessment and judgment.

- While transference requires only the appropriate signature, the approach depends on a careful investigation of published recommendations, access to appropriate information, and significant laboratory and medical experience to assure the comparability of conditions.

- Provision of reference intervals for sub-populations, particularly the pediatrics year-by-year intervals, often requires this approach because of the difficulty in obtaining sufficient specimens to experimentally establish or verify reference intervals.

2. Verification with 20 samples.

Experimental validation may be performed by collecting and analyzing specimens from 20 individuals who represent the reference sample population. If two or fewer test results fall outside the claimed or reported reference limits, the reference interval is considered verified, as illustrated in the figure.

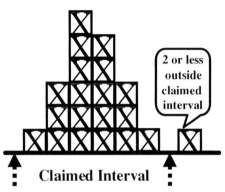

Verification with 20 samples

2 or less outside claimed interval

Claimed Interval

- Experimentally, this is a simple approach. It only requires a minimum of data, and the study provides a clear criterion for interpreting the data and verifying the transference.

- It is easiest to select the adult population, adult males, or adult females as the reference interval to verify, rather than a smaller sub-population.

3. Estimation with 60 samples.

An experimental validation may be performed by collecting and analyzing specimens from 60 individuals who represent the reference sample population. The actual reference interval is estimated and compared to the claimed or reported interval using a statistical formula comparing the means and standard deviations of the two populations [7].

- Sometimes finding even 60 reference individuals can be a daunting task. At the very least, no fewer than 40 individuals should be used to statistically calculate reference intervals. When fewer than 40 individuals are used, it is best to report the findings in terms of the minimum and maximum test values observed along with a histogram showing the distribution of the values.

- The statistical comparison of the observed and claimed or reported intervals is more complicated and therefore less attractive for verifying a reference interval than the 20-sample approach.

4. Calculation from comparative method.

The CLSI document also recognizes – but doesn't endorse – another approach that would adjust or correct the claimed or reported reference intervals on the basis of the observed methodological bias and the mathematical relationship demonstrated between the analytical methods being used (as shown in the figure at right). The regression statistics obtained from a comparison of methods study could be used to calculate the reference limits (X_{lower} and X_{upper}) to the new method ($Y_{lower} = a + bX_{lower}$, $Y_{upper} = a + bX_{upper}$, where a is the y-intercept and b is the slope of the regression line).

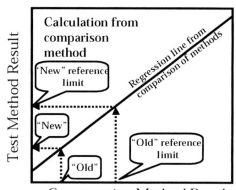

Comparative Method Result

- This approach is attractive when the laboratory has performed the studies necessary to establish its own reference intervals in the past and then changes to a new analytical method. In-house data should therefore be available to document the comparison of the new method with the old.

- Verification by analysis of 20 samples is recommended if there is any doubt about the reliability of the reference intervals being transferred from the comparative method.

- Transference by calculation should be limited to one changeover of methods to minimize the potential "cascade" of errors in setting new reference limits.

- This calculation approach is also advocated by Koivula [8] for transference of reference intervals from a reference laboratory to an individual laboratory. The laboratory analyzes six or seven carefully selected samples from an external quality assessment program and calculates the regression line between the values from the individual laboratory and the values from the reference laboratory. The reference interval from the reference laboratory is then used with the regression equation to calculate the reference limits for the individual laboratory.

What to do?

For tests where there are well-established reference intervals for the comparative method in your laboratory, transfer those intervals by calculation using the regression equation obtained from the comparison of methods experiment performed in your laboratory. Be sure the regression statistics are reliable by following the guidelines for performing the comparison of methods experiment and providing the proper statistical analysis of the data. Transference will require only a few additional calculations, making it quick and easy to determine the new limits. This approach should be suitable for common chemistry and hematology tests where one-to-one agreement can be expected.

For tests where there are systematic differences between the new and comparative methods, use the calculation approach, as above, to estimate the reference intervals and compare with the manufacturer's claims. Further verify the transferred limits by analysis of 20 specimens from healthy subjects. This approach would be appropriate with enzyme methods where proportional differences often exist between methods and immunoassays where systematic changes may occur between generations of measurement systems.

Use the 20 sample approach to transfer a manufacturer's recommendations when the manufacturer provides documentation of an adequate reference value study.

Use the 60 sample approach to make estimates of reference interval when the reference interval information from the manufacturer is not adequate, when the new test method is based on a different measurement principle and different measurement specificity, or when the test is being applied to a different patient population.

Use the divine judgment approach when there are no experimental data to support transference of the reference intervals.

References

1. Solberg HE. Approved recommendation (1986) on the theory of reference values. Part 1. The concept of reference values. Clin Chim Acta 1987;167:111-118.

2. PetitClerc C, Solberg HE. Approved recommendation (1987) on the theory of reference values. Part 2. Selection of individuals for the production of reference values. J Clin Chem Clin Biochem 1987;25:639-644.

3. Solberg HE, PetitClerc C. Approved recommendation (1988) on the theory of reference values. Part 3. Preparation of individuals and collection of specimens for the production of reference values. Clin Chim Acta 1988;177:S-S12.

4. Solberg HE, Stamm D. Approved recommendation on the theory of reference values. Part 4. Control of analytical variation in the production, transfer, and application of reference values. Eur J Clin Chem Clin Biochem 1991;29:531-535.

5. Solberg HE. Approved recommendations (1987) on the theory of reference values. Part 5. Statistical treatment of collected reference values. Determination of reference limits. J Clin Chem Clin Biochem 1987;25:656-656.

6. Dybkaer R, Solberg HE. Approved recommendations (1987) on the theory of reference values. Part 6. Presentation of observed values related to reference values. J Clin Chem Clin Biochem 1987;25:657-662.

7. CLSI C28-A2: How to define and determine reference intervals in the clinical laboratory - Second edition - Approved Guideline. Wayne, PA: Clinical Laboratory Standards Institute, 2000.

8. Koivula T. Possibilities for quality assurance of reference intervals. Scand J Clin Lab Invest 1995;55, Suppl. 222:17-20.

Self-Assessment Questions:

○ How many patient specimens are generally needed to *verify* a reference interval?

○ What is the minimum number of patient specimens to *establish* a reference interval?

○ How can a reference interval be *transferred* from the comparison method?

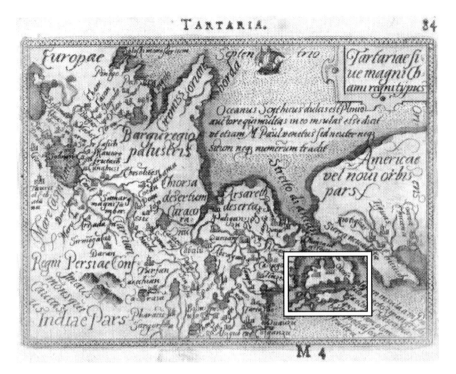

A note of caution about transference!
TARTARIAE SIVE MAGNI CHAMI REGNI TYPUS, by Philip Galle,
Antwerp, 1595.

This miniature of Ortelius's famous map of "Tartaria" illustrates
the mapmaker's "divine judgment" about the relationship between
Asia and America. Observe (in the lower right corner) that the
Island of Japan is almost equidistant between Asia and the California
peninsula of America. This map was constructed on the basis of
information about Asia and information about America, but without
any actual data on the size of the Pacific Ocean! In spite of the good
intention of the mapmaker, divine judgment resulted in a very
inaccurate description of the width of the Pacific Ocean and the
distance between Asia and America.

16: How do you judge the performance of a method?

You've performed the experiments, tabulated the results, plotted the data, and calculated the statistics. This chapter describes the next step, which is to make a judgment on the performance of the method. A graphical technique – the Method Decision Chart – is recommended and its construction and application are illustrated.

Objectives:

○ Construct a Method Decision Chart.

○ Evaluate the performance of a method using the Method Decision Chart.

○ Recommend appropriate action on the basis of the observed method performance.

Lesson materials:

○ **MV – The decision on method performance,**
   by James O. Westgard, PhD

○ **Method validation data analysis tool kit**
   http://www.westgard.com/mvtools.html

○ **Normalized operating point calculator**
   http://www.westgard.com/normcalc.htm

○ **Problem set: Cholesterol method validation data**

Things to do:

○ Study the materials.

○ Apply the Method Decision Chart to the cholesterol problem set.

○ Practice using the online calculators.

Method Validation:
The Decision on Method Performance

James O. Westgard, PhD

You've performed the experiments, tabulated the results, plotted the data, and calculated the statistics. Now you have to make a decision on the acceptability of the method. How do you decide whether the method is good enough to use in your laboratory?

What's the right approach?

Remember *The inner, hidden, deeper, secret, meaning* of method validation – ERROR ASSESSMENT. The decision on the acceptability of method performance depends on the size of the observed errors relative to some "standard" or quality requirement that defines the medically allowable error. Method performance is acceptable when the observed errors are smaller than the medically allowable error. Method performance is NOT acceptable when the observed errors are larger than the medically allowable error.

You should actually define the medically allowable errors at important medical decision levels in the beginning to help guide the design of the experiments and the collection of the data. What will remain to be done, then, is to compare your observed errors with the defined medically allowable errors.

How should a requirement for medically allowable errors be stated?

In the scientific literature, requirements for analytical quality have been defined in three different formats – allowable total error, allowable SD, and allowable bias. An allowable total error sets a limit on the combined effect of the random and systematic errors of a method, whereas an allowable SD and an allowable bias set separate limits for random and systematic errors, respectively.

Separate requirements for allowable SD and allowable bias would appear to be useful because these statistics can be calculated directly from the experimental data (e.g., an SD is calculated for the data from a replication experiment and a bias for the data from a comparison of methods experiment). However, the quality of a patient test result is determined by the net or total effect of both the random and systematic errors, therefore the total error is more relevant medically [1]:

> "The physician thinks rather in terms of the total analytical error, which includes both random and systematic components. From his point of view, all types of analytic error are acceptable as long as the total analytic error is less than a specified amount. Total error is medically more useful; after all, it makes little difference to the patient whether a laboratory value is in error because of random or systematic analytical error, and ultimately he is the one who must live with the error."

Where do you find recommendations for allowable total errors?

A common source is the external quality assessment survey or proficiency testing program in which you participate. These programs generally define a central "target value" and a range of values around that target that are considered acceptable. Because these programs usually ask for a single analysis on each survey specimen, both the random and systematic errors of your method will affect the results. The "acceptable range" is therefore an analytical performance requirement in the format of an allowable total error.

For US laboratories, the most readily available list of total error criteria are provided by the CLIA proficiency testing criteria for acceptable performance, which have been published in the Federal Register [2] and provide recommendations for over 70 different tests. See the list of criteria provided in Appendix 1. These criteria are presented in three different ways:

- As an absolute concentration limit, e.g., target value ± 1 mg/dL for calcium;
- As a percentage, e.g., target value ± 10% for albumin, cholesterol, and total protein;
- As the range determined from a survey group, e.g., target value ± 3 standard deviations for thyroid stimulating hormone.

In a few cases, two sets of limits are given, e.g., the glucose requirement is target value ± 6 mg/dL or ± 10%, whichever is greater. At a medical decision level of 50 mg/dL, the allowable total error is 6 mg/dL or 12%. At a medical decision level of 125 mg/dL, the allowable total error is 10% or 12.5 mg/dL.

How are the observed errors compared to a total allowable error?

To estimate the random error of the method from the replication experiment, you will calculate an SD or CV. To estimate systematic error from the comparison of methods experiment, you will calculate the bias between the means obtained by the test and comparative methods, or use regression statistics to calculate the expected difference at particular medical decision levels. These estimates of random and systematic errors need to be combined to judge their total effect.

The literature provides four different recommendations on how to combine random and systematic errors:

- Add bias + 2 times the observed SD [ref 1], i.e., bias + 2SD < TE_a;
- Add bias + 3 times the observed SD [ref 3], i.e., bias + 3SD < TE_a;
- Add bias + 4 times the observed SD [ref 4], i.e., bias + 4SD < TE_a;
- Add bias + 6 times the observed SD [ref 5], i.e., bias + 5SD < TE_a.

Rather than choose between these recommendations, all can be incorporated into a graphical decision tool – a Method Decision Chart [6]. The chart is simple to construct, minimizes the need for additional calculations, and provides a graphical picture that simplifies the interpretation and judgment on method performance.

How do you construct a Method Decision Chart?

First, express the allowable total error as a percentage of the medical decision concentration. Most CLIA allowable errors are already given this way. For those given in concentration units, express the allowable error as a percent of the medical decision concentration of interest, i.e., divide the allowable error by the medical decision concentration and multiply by 100 to express as a percentage.

Next, take a sheet of graph paper and do the following:

1. Label the y-axis "Allowable inaccuracy, (bias,%)" and scale from 0 to TE_a, e.g., for $TE_a = 10\%$, scale the y-axis from 0 to 10% in increments of 1%.

2. Label the x-axis "Allowable imprecision, (s,%) and scale from 0 to 0.5 TE_a, e.g., for $TE_a = 10\%$, scale the x-axis from 0 to 5% in increments of 0.5%.

3. Draw a line for bias + 2 SD from TE_a on the y-axis to 0.5 TE_a on the x-axis, e.g., for $TE_a = 10\%$, draw the line from 10% (y-axis) to 5% (x-axis).

4. Draw a line for bias + 3 SD from TE_a on the y-axis to 0.33 TE_a on the x-axis, e.g., for $TE_a = 10\%$, draw the line from 10% (y-axis) to 3.33% (x-axis).

5. Draw a line for bias + 4 SD from TE_a on the y-axis to 0.25 TE_a on the x-axis, e.g., for $TE_a = 10\%$, draw the line from 10% (y-axis) to 2.5% (x-axis).

6. Draw a line for bias + 5 SD from TE_a on the y-axis to 0.20 TE_a on the x-axis, e.g., for $TE_a = 10\%$, draw the line from 10% (y-axis) to 2.0% (x-axis).

7. Draw a line for bias + 6 SD from TE_a on the y-axis to 0.17 TE_a on the x-axis, e.g., for $TE_a = 10\%$, draw the line from 10% (y-axis) to 1.7% (x-axis).

8. Label the regions "unacceptable", "poor," "marginal," "good," "excellent," and "world class" as shown in the figure.

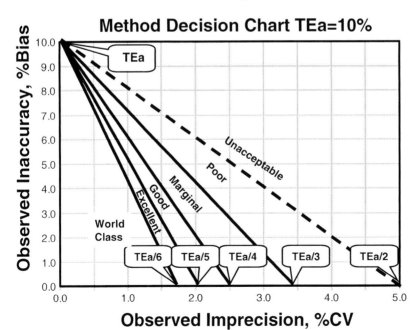

How do you use the Method Decision Chart?

Express your observed SD and bias in percent, then plot the point whose x-coordinate is your observed imprecision and y-coordinate is your observed inaccuracy. This point is called the "operating point" because it describes how your method operates. You judge the performance of your method on the basis of the location of the operating point, as follows:

- A method with **unacceptable performance** does not meet your requirement for quality, even when the method is working properly. It is not acceptable for routine operation.

- A method with **poor performance** might have been considered acceptable prior to the recent introduction of the principles of Six Sigma Quality Management, but industrial benchmarks now set a minimum standard of 3-Sigma performance for a routine production process, thus performance in the region between 2-Sigma and 3-Sigma is not really satisfactory today.

- A method with **marginal performance** provides the necessary quality when everything is working correctly. However, it will be difficult to manage in routine operation, will require 4 to 8 controls per run, and a Total QC strategy that emphasizes well-trained operators, reduced rotation of personnel, more aggressive preventive maintenance, careful monitoring of patient test results, and continual efforts to improve method performance.

- A method with **good performance** meets your requirement for quality and can be well-managed in routine operation with 2 to 4 control measurements per run using multirule QC procedures or a single control rule having 2.5s control limits.

- A method with **excellent performance** is clearly acceptable and can be well-managed in routine operation with only 2 control measurements per run using a single control rule with 2.5s or 3.0s control limits.

- A method with **world class performance** is even easier to manage and control, usually requiring only 1 or 2 control measurements per run and a single control rule with wide limits, such as 3.0s or 3.5s.

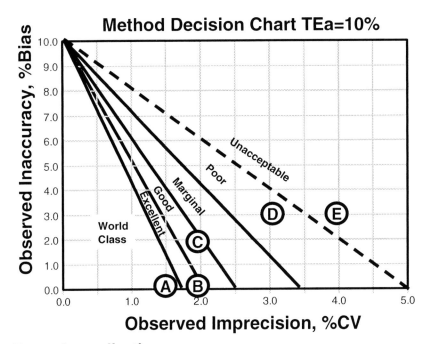

Method Decision Chart TEa=10%

Example applications

All these examples illustrate the evaluation of cholesterol methods, where the CLIA requirement for acceptable performance is an allowable total error of 10%

A. A cholesterol method with a CV of 1.5% and a bias of 0.0% provides world class quality, as shown by the operating point labeled A, whose x-coordinate is 1.5 and y-coordinate is 0.0. This method is clearly acceptable and will be easy to manage and control in routine operation using 2 control measurements per run and a single control rule having 3.5s control limits.

B. A cholesterol method with a CV of 2.0% and bias of 0.0% provides excellent performance, as shown by operating point B. This method is clearly acceptable and will be controllable in routine service using 2 control measurements and a single control rule having 3.0s or 2.5s control limits.

C. A cholesterol method with a CV of 2.0% and a bias of 2.0% has an operating point that falls on the line between good performance and marginal performance, as shown by point C. A careful assessment of QC is required and will show that a multirule procedure with a total of 4 control measurements per run is necessary to guarantee the desired quality for this method [7]. See also the QC application on Westgard Web at http://www.westgard.com/qcapp3.htm.

D. A cholesterol method having a CV of 3.0% and a bias of 3.0% satisfies the specifications of the National Cholesterol Education Program (NCEP) [7]. To assess whether these performance specifications are adequate, an operating point can be ploted with a y-coordinate of 3.0% and an x-coordinate of 3.0%, as shown by the point labeled D in the accompanying figure. Such a method has poor performance and will only achieve the desired quality *if everything is working perfectly*. It will be very difficult to detect problems and maintain the desired quality during routine service [Note that we disagree with the CDC on the methodology that is appropriate for setting performance specifications. Reference 8 provides some discussion and debate. Reference 9 is an expansive defense of the CDC-NCEP methodology.]

E. A cholesterol method with a CV of 4.0% and a bias of 3.0% may be representative of the type of screening methods encountered in shopping malls and pharmacies. As shown by operating point E, such a method does not provide the quality necessary to meet the CLIA requirement for acceptable performance *even if everything is working perfectly.*

Try it!

Define the allowable total error for your test. Construct a Method Decision Chart using a page of graph paper. Plot your observed inaccuracy (% bias) from the comparison of methods experiment versus the observed imprecision (% s or CV) from the replication experiment. See where this operating point is located and judge whether or not you want to implement the method for routine service.

Try it with Online Calculators!

On Westgard Web, two tools are available:

Method Decision Calculator
http://www.westgard.com/mvtools.html

Normalized Operating Point Calculator
http://www.westgard.com/normcalc.htm .

The Method Decision Calculator works by sending your entered values back to the server for calculation and preparation of the Method Decision Chart. The Normalized Operating Point Calculator is a Javascript calculator that performs the calculations on your computer. However, it can't prepare a graph so you need to print the accompanying Normalized Method Decision Chart and manually plot your operating point.

An automated Method Decision Chart is also available on Westgard Web – as a Excel spreadsheet file. You can download the file at http://www.westgard.com/medxcel.htm

References:

1. Westgard JO, Carey RN, Wold S. Criteria for judging precision and accuracy in method development and evaluation. Clin Chem 1974;20:825-33.

2. U.S. Department of Health and Social Services. Medicare, Medicaid, and CLIA Programs: Regulations implementing the Clinical Laboratory Improvement Amendments of 1988 (CLIA). Final Rule. Fed Regist 1992(Feb 28);57:7002-7186.

3. Ehrmeyer SS, Laessig RH, Leinweber JE, Oryall JE. 1990 Medicare/CLIA final rules for proficiency testing: Minimum interlaboratory performance characteristics (CV and Bias) needed to pass. Clin Chem 1990;36:1736-40.

4. Westgard JO, Burnett RW. Precision requirements for cost-effective operation of analytical processes. Clin Chem 1990;36:1629-32.

5. Westgard JO. Six Sigma Quality Design and Control, 2nd Edition, Chapter 7. Madison WI: Westgard QC, Inc., 2006, pp.91-105.

6. Westgard JO. A method evaluation decision chart (MEDx Chart) for judging method performance. Clin Lab Science. 1995;8:277-83.

7.   Westgard JO, Wiebe DA. Cholesterol operational process specifications for assuring the quality required by CLIA proficiency testing. Clin Chem 1991;37:1938-44.

8.   Westgard JO, Wiebe DA. Adequacy of NCEP recommendations for total cholesterol, triglycerides, HDLC, and LDLC measurements. Clin Chem 1998;44:1064-1066.

9.   Caudill SP, Cooper GR, Smith SJ, Myers GL. Assessment of current National Cholesterol Education Program guidelines for total cholesterol, triglycerides, HDL-cholesterol, and LDL-cholesterol measurements. Clin Chem 1998;44:1650-8.

Online References:

A method evaluation decision chart (MEDx) for judging method performance. Original paper in PDF format.
http://www.westgard.com/medx.htm

Method Decision calculator
http://www.westgard.com/mvtools.html

Method Decision Chart Excel spreadsheet
http://www.westgard.com/medxcel.htm

Normalized operating point calculator
http://www.westgard.com/normcalc.htm

Self-Assessment Questions:

○ How is a quality requirement incorporated into a Method Decision Chart?

○ What's a common source of quality requirement for a test?

○ What critical performance parameters are plotted on a Method Decision Chart?

○ What are the performance classifications on a Method Decision Chart?

○ What is your judgment on a calcium method whose observed SD is 0.2 mg/dL and observed bias is 0.1 mg/dL at a decision level of 11.0?

17: What's a practical procedure for validating a method?

This chapter reviews the overall approach to method validation and provides a set of worksheets for collecting the minimum amounts of data needed in each experiment. Following this approach and using these worksheets, you can plan and organize your own method validation study.

Objectives:

- ○ Review the overall approach to method validation.

- ○ Develop worksheets for collecting the appropriate experimental data.

- ○ Organize these worksheets into a practical method validation plan.

- ○ Determine the statistical support needed to implement a method validation plan.

Lesson materials:

- ○ **MV – The real world applications,** by James O. Westgard, PhD

- ○ **MV – The worksheets**

Things to do:

- ○ Study the materials.

- ○ Adapt the worksheets to fit your own needs.

Method Validation:
The Real World Applications

James O. Westgard, PhD

The previous chapters provided you with the skills to establish your own method validation process. It is important to establish a systematic process that is tailored to the needs of your laboratory and to the characteristics of the methods being tested. Don't assume that method performance is okay just because you've purchased new instrument or new reagent kit! In the real world, methods still have problems. Remember the *Myths of quality*?

A review of the MV process

Here's a brief summary of our lessons on method validation. You can review the earlier chapters for further detail and clarification of the major points.

- Method Validation should be a standard laboratory process, but the process need not be exactly the same for every laboratory or for every method validated by a laboratory. See *Management of Quality – The need for standard processes and standards of quality* for an overview of the quality management process that is needed in healthcare laboratories and the role of method validation in establishing standard testing processes.

- Remember the purpose of method validation is error assessment. See *The inner, hidden, deeper, secret meaning* for a description of random, systematic, and total analytical errors that are the focus of method validation studies.

- Note that a US laboratory is required by CLIA regulations to "demonstrate that prior to reporting patient test results, it can obtain the performance specifications for accuracy, precision, and reportable range of patient test results, comparable to those established by the manufacturer. The laboratory must also verify that the manufacturer's reference range is appropriate for the laboratory's patient population."

For non-waived methods, CLIA also requires verification of analytical sensitivity and analytical specificity. See *The regulations.*

- Other critical method factors or characteristics, such as cost/ test, specimen types, specimen volumes, time required for analysis, rate of analysis, equipment required, personnel required, efficiency, safety, etc., must be considered during the selection of the analytical method. See *Selecting a method to validate.*

- The approach in method validation is to perform a series of experiments designed to estimate certain types of analytical errors, e.g., a linearity experiment to determine reportable range, a replication experiment to estimate imprecision or random error, a comparison of methods experiment to estimate inaccuracy or systematic error, or interference and recovery experiments to specifically estimate constant and proportional systematic errors (analytical specificity), and a detection limit experiment to characterize analytical sensitivity. See *The experimental plan.* For details of the different types of experiments, see the following:

  - *The linearity or reportable range experiment.* A minimum of 5 specimens with known or assigned values should be analyzed in triplicate to assess the reportable range.

  - *The replication experiment.* A minimum of 20 replicate determinations on at least two levels of control materials are recommended to estimate the imprecision or random error of the method.

  - *The comparison of methods experiment.* A minimum of 40 patient specimens should be analyzed by the new method (test method) and an established method (comparison method) to estimate the inaccuracy or systematic error of the method.

  - *The interference and recovery experiments.* Common interferences, such as lipemia, hemolysis, and elevated bilirubin are usually tested, along with potential interferences that are specific to the test and methodology. Recovery experiments are used to test competitive interferences, such as the possible effects of proteins and metabolics in the specimens.

- *The detection limit experiment.* The detection limit is determined for those methods whose low test values are critically interpreted. Generally, a "blank" specimen and a specimen "spiked" with the amount of analyte in the manufacturer's claim for the limit of detection are each analyzed 20 times.

- The data collected in the different experiments needs to be summarized (by statistical calculations) to provide estimates of the analytical errors that are the focus of each experiment. See *The data analysis tool kit.*

- The acceptability of these observed errors is judged by comparison to standards of quality, i.e., recommendations for the allowable total error such as provided by the CLIA proficiency testing criteria. Method performance is acceptable when the observed errors are smaller than the stated limits of allowable error. A graphical tool – the Method Decision Chart – can be used to classify performance as world class (Six Sigma), excellent, good, marginal, poor, or unacceptable. [1] See *The decision on method performance.*

- If method performance is judged acceptable, the reference intervals should be verified. See *Reference Interval Transference.*

Applications with published data

A critical review of the literature is always a good starting point when selecting and evaluating a method. This can include scientific papers as well as the manufacturer's method descriptions. The time and effort needed for method validation studies in your own laboratory can be minimized by a careful assessment of the data in the literature.

Published validation studies seldom follow a standard validation process. Therefore, it is necessary to impose your own system of organization, data analysis, and data interpretation if you want to make sense of the results. This is a process of critical review, which is distinctly different from just accepting the format, data analysis, and conclusions that have been published.

- Define the quality requirement in the form of an allowable total error (TE_a) for the test (or tests) of interest at the medical decision concentration for critical test interpretation. Note that few journals require the authors to declare the quality that they consider acceptable, therefore the conclusions of many published studies rarely refer to any standards of quality. The notable exception is the journal *Clinical Chemistry* which began in January 1999 to advise contributors that they should reference their method performance findings to defined quality standards [2]. Alas, few papers follow that advice.

- Prepare a "data page" to summarize information about the experiments. List the standard experiments that would be expected, e.g., reportable range, within-day replication, day-to-day replication, interference, recovery, and comparison of methods.

- Scan the published report to locate the different experiments, summarize the critical factors (number of patient specimens, number of replicate measurements, etc), and identify the strengths and weaknesses of the published studies.

  - For a *replication experiment*, assess the suitability of the concentrations of the control materials, the sample matrix, the time period of study, and other conditions, such as the number of different reagent lots included, number of analysts involved, etc. Tabulate the number of measurements, the mean, and the standard deviation or coefficient of variation for each material.

  - For an *interference experiment*, assess whether the substances and concentrations tested are appropriate. Tabulate the average difference or bias as your estimate of constant systematic error.

- For a *recovery experiment*, determine how the calculations were done (whether recovery was calculated on the total amount measured or on the amount added, the latter being the correct way). Tabulate the number of experiments and the average recovery. Calculate the proportional error (100 – average %Recovery), then multiply times the critical medical decision concentrations to estimate the proportional systematic error.

- For a *detection limit experiment*, clarify the definition of the particular term being used and the experimental approach for making the estimate. Identify the samples analyzed, the number of replicate measurements, and the equation for calculating the detection limit.

- For a *comparison experiment*, assess whether the comparison method itself is a good choice. Tabulate the number of patient specimens analyzed by the two methods, the concentration range studied, and the distribution of data over that range. Tabulate the statistics results (most likely t-test and regression statistics). Assess whether linear regression statistics will provide reliable estimates of errors by inspecting a comparison plot and also from the value of the correlation coefficient (which should be 0.99 or higher). When regression statistics are reliable, estimate the inaccuracy or systematic error from the equation $SE = (a + bX_c) - X_c$, where a is the y-intercept, b is the slope, and X_c is the critical medical decision concentration. If ordinary regression statistics do not provide reliable estimates of errors, determine whether the bias from t-test statistics will be reliable, which requires that the mean of the comparison results must be close to the medical decision concentration of interest.

- Use the Method Decision Chart to assess whether method performance is satisfactory for your laboratory. Show the individual estimates of systematic errors or inaccuracy (from interference and recovery experiments) as points on the y-axis; show the individual estimates of random errors or imprecision as points on the x-axis. Assess the combined effects of random and systematic errors by plotting the operating point whose y-coordinate is the bias or SE from the comparison of methods experiment and whose x-coordinate is the CV from the day-to-day replication study.

- Review the authors' conclusions and recommendations. Resolve any differences between your conclusions and those of the authors. Identify the factors that will be critical if you test the method in your own laboratory.

Applications in your own laboratory

It is important to have a clear understanding of the method validation process and be well-organized in carrying out your experimental studies. Good record keeping is essential to document the conditions of the studies (reagent lot numbers, calibration lot numbers, re-calibrations, preventive maintenance procedures, any method changes or corrective actions).

- Carefully specify the application, methodology, and performance requirements for the test of interest. State the quality requirement for the test in the form of an allowable total error (TE_a), such as specified in many proficiency testing programs. Conduct a careful literature search and select a method that has appropriate application and methodology characteristics and has a good chance of achieving the desired performance.

- Develop a validation plan on the basis of the characteristics of the test and method that will be critical for its successful application in your laboratory. Identify the experiments, specify the amount of data to be collected, and identify the decision concentrations or analytical ranges where the data should be collected. Schedule personnel time to carry out the validation studies.

- Implement the method validation plan by preparing a set of worksheets that define the amount of data to be collected in the different experiments. These worksheets will formalize the planning of the experiments and also facilitate the collection of the data.

- The *reportable range worksheet* should have columns for the date, analyst, sample identification, assigned or known value, observed result #1, observed result #2, observed result #3, average result, and comments. The number of rows will depend on the number of specimens analyzed, which will usually be from 5 to 10. Also include information about the source of the specimens, preparation of specimen pools, manufacturer and lot numbers of commercial materials. See page 207.

- The *replication worksheet* should have columns for date, time, analyst, result for material 1, result for material 2, (result for material 3 if needed), and comments. The number of rows should be a minimum of 20. Also include information about the manufacturer and the lot numbers for the control materials being analyzed. Note that you will usually need one worksheet for the within-day replication study and a second for the day-to-day study. See page 208.

- The *comparison of methods worksheet* should have columns for date, analyst, specimen identification number, test result (y-value), comparison result (x-value), difference (y-x), and comments. Add extra columns if duplicate measurements are to be performed. The number of rows should be 40. See page 209-210.

- Begin plotting the comparison data on a daily basis as it is collected. Identify discrepant values and repeat those tests by both methods. A difference plot will point out these discrepancies more clearly than a comparison plot, but either or both can be used for this purpose.

- Perform the statistical calculations that are appropriate for the data collected in the different experiments.

- Use the Medical Decision Chart to assess whether method performance is satisfactory for your laboratory.

- Document the method validation studies. If method performance is acceptable, prepare a method procedure to document the standard testing process. Prepare teaching materials for in-service training. Select appropriate QC materials, control rules, and numbers of control measurements to monitor routine performance.

Adaptations for individual laboratory applications

It should be recognized that each laboratory situation may be different, therefore, different adaptations are possible in different laboratories. The approach we advocate is to maintain the principles of the method validation process, while making the experimental work as efficient and practical as possible. Some ideas are presented here concerning the scope of studies, personnel skills, and data analysis techniques.

- The scope of studies may be adapted on the basis of the information available in the scientific literature. Minimal work can be performed when thorough studies have been published. Always perform a linearity or reportable range experiment and a replication study over at least ten days. Reduce the number of patient comparisons to 20 specimens whose concentrations are selected to span the analytical range. Minimize the use of recovery and interference studies. Likewise, when replacing a method or instrument with the same or similar method or instrument, your earlier laboratory experience allows you to reduce the amount of data needed to validate the new method or instrument.

- New technology or changes in method or measurement principles will require more extensive validation studies. New methodology that is just being released and not yet in widespread use must be critically evaluated. If the laboratory is involved in "field testing" for a manufacturer, even more extensive studies will be required, way beyond the minimums suggested here for basic method validation studies.

- The laboratory personnel involved in method validation studies may have a variety of experience. However, it is important to have at least one skilled analyst to organize the studies, specify the amount of data to be collected, monitor the data during collection to identify obvious method problems, carefully inspect the data to identify discrepant results, properly analyze the data statistically, critically interpret the results, and make any necessary changes or adjustments to the validation plan. Other analysts may carry out the experiments and tabulate the data. Participation of several analysts will provide more realistic estimates of the imprecision expected under routine operation of the method.

- The data analysis should be understandable by the laboratory analysts, otherwise good data may still not provide good decisions about method performance. The comparison of methods data are the most difficult to analyze. A plot of the data should always be prepared. Regression statistics are generally preferred, but t-test statistics may be sufficient when the estimate of bias is obtained at a mean that is very close to the medical decision level of interest. See chapters 8, 12, and 18 for more detailed guidelines on the data analysis.

References

1. Westgard JO. A method evaluation decision chart (MEDx) Chart for judging method performance. Clin Lab Science 1995;8:277-83. See below for PDF files.

2. Information for authors. Journal of Clinical Chemistry http://www.clinchem.org/info_ar/anal_meth.shtml

Online References:

A method evaluation decision chart for judging method performance. http://www.westgard.com/medx.htm

Method Decision Chart spreadsheet http://www.westgard.com/medxcel.htm

Points of Care in using statistics in method comparison studies. http://www.westgard.com/essay19.htm

Self-Assessment Questions:

○ What are the minimum experiments needed for your tests?

○ What is the minimum number of measurements needed for each experiment?

○ What is the best organization of these experiments?

○ What is the most practical way to make the data calculations?

Reportable Range Experiment

Test: _____

Method: _____

Materials: _____

#	Date	Analyst	Sample ID	Assigned Value	Result 1	Result 2	Result 3	Average	Comments
1									
2									
3									
4									
5									
6									

Replication Experiment

Test: _____
Method: _____
Materials: _____

#	Date	Time	Analyst	Material 1 Result	Material 2 Result	Material 3 Result	Comments
1							
2							
3							
4							
5							
6							
7							
8							
9							
10							
11							
12							
13							
14							
15							
16							
17							
18							
19							
20							

Comparison Experiment
Part I

Test: _____
Method: _____
Comp. Method: _____

#	Date	Analyst	Specimen ID#	Test Result(y)	Comparison Result (x)	Diff (y-x)	Comments
1							
2							
3							
4							
5							
6							
7							
8							
9							
10							
11							
12							
13							
14							
15							
16							
17							
18							
19							
20							

Comparison Experiment Part II

Test: _____

Method: _____

Comp. Method: _____

#	Date	Analyst	Specimen ID#	Test Result(y)	Comparison Result (x)	Diff (y-x)	Comments
21							
22							
23							
24							
25							
26							
27							
28							
29							
30							
31							
32							
33							
34							
35							
36							
37							
38							
39							
40							

18: How do you use statistics in the Real World?

This chapter provides one last dose of statistics. Most students learn statistics slowly, a few ideas at a time. It takes many doses to build up a person's knowledge of statistics and their skills in applying and interpreting statistics correctly. Sometimes it is a matter of hearing or seeing the information presented in a different way. Here's another way of working through the proper use and interpretation of statistics in method comparison studies.

Objectives:

- Review the use of statistics in method comparison studies.
- Summarize the important considerations for proper use of regression statistics.
- Identify when to use more sophisticated regression techniques, such as Deming regression and Passing-Bablock regression.

Lesson materials:

- **Points of care in using statistics in method comparison studies**, by James O. Westgard, PhD

Things to do:

- Study the materials.
- Review a published validation study and critique the application of statistics.

Some Points-of-Care in using statistics in method validation

This is an updated and annotated version of an editorial that appeared in the 1998 November issue of Clinical Chemistry, volume 44, pages 2240-2242.

James O. Westgard, PhD

As clinical chemists and laboratory scientists, we are often concerned when personnel who have little laboratory training begin to perform laboratory tests, such as point-of-care applications. It may be easy to perform such tests today with modern analytical systems, but there still are things that can go wrong. We hope that some kind of quality system is used to check that everything is working correctly with point-of-care analyses.

Imagine how statisticians feel about the powerful statistics programs that are now in our hands. It's so easy to key-in a set of data and calculate a wide variety of statistics – regardless of what those statistics are or what they mean. There is a need to check that things are done correctly in the statistical analyses we perform in our laboratories.

In the November 1998 issue of *Clinical Chemistry*, Stockl, Dewitte, and Thienpont [1] pointed out that the quality of the data may be more important than the quality of the regression technique (e.g., ordinary linear regression vs Deming regression vs Passing-Bablock regression). In the journal *Clinical Chemistry*, the standard method for analyzing the data from a method com-

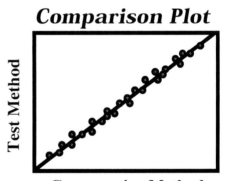

Comparison Plot

Test Method (y-axis) / Comparative Method (x-axis)

parison experiment has been to prepare a *comparison plot* that shows the test method results on the y-axis and the comparative method results on the x-axis, then calculate regression statistics to determine the best line of fit for the data. Different regression techniques may be appropriate, depending on the characteristics of the data – particularly the analytical range that is covered relative to the test values that are critical for medical applications.

Elsewhere in the literature [2], there is a movement to discourage the use of regression analysis altogether and replace it with a simple graphical presentation of method-comparison data in the form of a *difference plot*, which displays the difference between the test and comparative results on the y-axis vs the mean of the test and comparative results on the x-axis. This difference plot has become known as the Bland-Altman plot [3]. Hyltoft-Petersen et al [4] have shown that a difference plot must be carefully constructed to make an objective decision about method performance. The difference plot is actually not so simple when an objective interpretation is to be made.

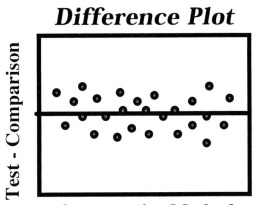

Difference Plot

Test - Comparison

Comparative Method

In spite of these recent reports and recommendations on the use of statistics, many analysts and investigators still have difficulties with method comparison data. We studied some of the problems over thirty years ago [5]. For the most part, there are similar problems today – with the exception that the calculations are much easier to perform with today's computer programs. There has not been much improvement, if any, in the basic statistical knowledge and skills available in laboratories today, not only for method validation studies but also for statistical quality control. That doesn't mean there haven't been improvements in the theory and recommendations appearing in the literature, but rather that the practices in laboratories really haven't changed.

Therefore, we still need to exercise a great deal of care in collecting, analyzing, and interpreting method comparison data. Here are some points to be careful about:

Point #1: Use statistics to provide estimates of errors, not as indicators of acceptability. This is perhaps the most fundamental point for making practical sense of statistics in method validation studies. Remember that the purpose of a method validation study is to estimate or validate claims for method performance characteristics. [See *The inner, hidden, deeper, secret meaning.*] Application and methodology characteristics should be dealt with during the selection of the method. [See *Selecting a method to validate.*] The statistics are simply tools for quantitating the size of the errors from data collected in different method validation experiments. [See *The data analysis tool kit.*]

The statistics don't directly tell you whether the method is acceptable, rather they provide *estimates of errors* which allow you to judge the acceptability of a method. You do this by comparing the amount of error observed with the amount of error that would be allowable without compromising the medical use and interpretation of the test result. Method performance is judged acceptable when the observed error is smaller than the defined allowable error. Method performance is not acceptable when the observed error is larger than the allowable error. This decision-making process can be facilitated by mathematical criteria [6] or by graphic tools [7]. [See *The decision on method performance.*]

Point #2: Recognize that the main purpose of the method comparison experiment is to obtain an estimate of systematic error or bias. The comparison of methods experiment is performed to study the accuracy of a new method. [See *The experimental plan.*] The essential information is the average systematic error, or bias. It is also useful to obtain information about the proportional and constant nature of the systematic error and to quantify the random error between the methods. The components of error are important because they relate to the things we can manage in the laboratory to control the total error of the testing process (e.g., reduce proportional systematic error by improved calibration). The total error is important in judging the acceptability of a method and can be calculated from the components.

Point #3: Obtain estimates of systematic error at important medical decision concentrations. The collection of specimens and choice of statistics can be optimized by focusing on the concentration (or concentrations) where the interpretation of a test result will be most critical for the medical application of the test. [See the summary of *medical decision levels* by Dr. Bernard Statland] If there is only a single medical decision concentration, the method comparison data may be collected around that level (i.e., a wide range of data will not be necessary) and a difference plot should be useful (along with an estimate of bias from t-test analysis – see point #8 below). If there are two or more decision levels, it is desirable to collect specimens that cover a wide analytical range, use a comparison plot to display the results, and calculate regression statistics to estimate the systematic error at each of the decision levels.

Point #4: When there is a single medical decision level, make the estimate of systematic error near the mean of the data. The main consideration when there is a single medical decision level is to collect the data around that medical decision level. The choice of statistics will not be critical when there is only one medical decision level of interest and it falls near the mean of the data. The bias statistic from paired t-test calculations and the systematic error calculated from regression statistics will provide the same estimate of the error.

[Note of explanation: The bias is the difference between the means of the two methods (bias = $Y_{av} - X_{av}$), which is also equivalent to the average of the paired differences from paired t-test calculations. With regression statistics, the systematic error (SE) is estimated at a critical concentration, X_c, as follows: SE = $Y_c - X_c$, where Y_c is calculated from the regression statistics by the equation $Y_c = a + bX_c$, where a is the y-intercept and b is the slope of the regression line. In ordinary linear regression, the slope is calculated first, then the y-intercept is determined from $a = Y_{av} - bX_{av}$. When the decision concentration equals X_{av}, then $SE = (a + bX_{av}) - X_{av} = Y_{av} - bX_{av} + bX_{av} - X_{av} = Y_{av} - X_{av}$, i.e., the same estimate of systematic error will be obtained from regression statistics as from t-test statistics, even if the range of data is narrow and the values for the slope and intercept are not reliable.]

Point #5: When there are two or more medical decision levels, use the correlation coefficient, r, to assess whether the range of data is adequate for using ordinary regression analysis. As confirmed by Stockl, Dewitte, and Thienpont [1], when r is 0.99 or greater, the range of data should be wide enough for ordinary linear regression to provide reliable estimates of the slope and intercept. They recommend that when r is less than 0.975, ordinary linear regression may not be reliable and that data improvement or alternate statistics are now appropriate. Note that r is *not* used to judge the acceptability of method performance, but is only used to judge the acceptability of the concentration range of the data being used to calculate the regression statistics.

Point #6. When r is high, use the comparison plot along with ordinary linear regression statistics. The reliability of the slope and intercept are affected by outliers and non-linearity, as well as the concentration range of the data [5]. Outliers need to be identified, preferably at the time of analysis by immediately plotting the data on the comparison graph; discrepant results can then be investigated while the specimens are still available. Non-linearity can usually be identified from visual inspection of the comparison plot, the range can be restricted to the linear portion, and the statistics recalculated. Stockl, Dewitte, and Thienpont [1] recommend using the residual plot that is available as part of regression analysis and inspecting the sign-sequence of the residuals for making this assessment.

Point #7: When r is low, improve the data or change the statistical technique. Consider the alternatives of improving the range of data, reducing the variation from the comparison method by replicate analyses, estimating the systematic error at the mean of the data, dividing the data into subgroups whose means agree with the medical decision levels (which can then be analyzed by t-test statistics and the difference plot), or using a more complicated regression technique. Stockl, Dewitte, and Thienpont find that the Deming regression technique is more satisfactory than the Passing-Bablock technique. Note that these regression techniques are not standard in ordinary statistics programs, but they are available in special programs designed for laboratory method validation studies.

Point #8: When r is low and a difference plot is used, calculate t-test statistics to provide a quantitative estimate of systematic error. Given the objective of estimating systematic error from the method comparison experiment, the usefulness of the difference plot by itself is questionable since visual interpretation will be mainly influenced by the scatter or random error observed between the methods. The bias, or average difference of paired sample results, should be calculated. Computer routines for calculating t-test statistics will provide this estimate, along with an estimate of the standard deviation of the differences, which gives a quantitative measure of the scatter between the methods. Note that this scatter between the methods depends on the imprecision of the test method, the imprecision of the comparison method, and any interferences that affect individual samples differently by the two methods. The t-value itself is a ratio of systematic to random error, and is mainly useful for determining if sufficient data has been collected to make a reliable estimate of the bias (again, avoid using a statistic as an indicator of the acceptability of the method). While Bland-Altman also recommend calculation of the mean difference and the standard deviation of the differences and suggest that the mean difference ± 2 standard deviations be drawn on the chart [3], it is wrong to judge the acceptability of the observed differences by comparison to themselves. See Hyltoft-Petersen et al [4] for an extensive discussion of judging method acceptability on the basis of the difference plot.

Point #9. When in doubt about the validity of the statistical technique, see whether the choice of statistics changes the outcome or decision on acceptability. Given the ease with which the calculations can be performed with computer programs, the effect of the statistical technique on the estimates of performance can be assessed by comparing the results from the different techniques. If the statistical technique affects your decision on the acceptability of the method, then be careful. Usually it will be best to collect more data and be sure these new data satisfy the assumptions of the data analysis technique.

Point #10: Plan the experiment carefully and collect the data appropriate for the statistical technique to be used. You can collect the data to fit the assumptions of the statistics, or you can change the statistics to compensate for limitations in the data. An understanding of the proper use and application of the statistics will help you plan the experiment and minimize the difficulties in interpreting the results. [See *The comparison of methods experiment.*] If you are establishing a standard method validation process in your laboratory, it may be best to put your efforts into collecting the appropriate data – my personal recommendation as the best approach for most healthcare laboratories. This emphasis on getting good data also involves collecting the right specimens under the right conditions, processing those specimens properly, storing the samples appropriately, operating the method or analytical system under representative conditions, and analyzing the patient samples with a process that is under statistical control. This point requires the most care and should have the highest priority. The statistics really don't matter if you don't take care with the data.

In quality management terms, the proper use of statistics is a chronic problem that will continue to flare up until the process is fixed. The process that needs fixing here is the education and training process in clinical chemistry, clinical pathology, and clinical laboratory science. There's a deficiency in a core competency – the ability to use basic statistics in method validation studies as well as for statistical quality control. Correcting this deficiency requires courses for students in undergraduate programs, continuing education workshops and seminars for professionals already in the field, and periodic articles in the scientific literature to remind investigators of the problems and difficulties. With today's Internet, basic training courses and software tools can be delivered to anyone, anywhere, anytime.

References

1. Stockl D, Dewitte K, Thienpont M. Validity of linear regression in method comparison studies: limited by the statistical model or the quality of the analytical data? Clin Chem 1998;44:2340-6.

2. Hollis S. Analysis of method comparison studies [editorial]. Ann Clin Biochem 1996;33:1-4.

3. Bland JM, Altman DG. Statistical methods for assessing agreement beween two methods of clinical measurement. Lancet 1986;307-10.

4. Hyltoft-Petersen P, Stockl D, Blaabjerg O, Pedersen B, Birkemose E, Thienpont L, Flensted Lassen J, Kjeldsen J. Graphical interpretration of analytical data from comparison of a field method with a reference method by use of difference plots [opinion]. Clin Chem 1997;43:2039-46.

5. Westgard JO, Hunt MR. Use and interpretation of common statistical tests in method-comparison studies. Clin Chem 1973;19:49-57. See below for PDF files.

6. Westgard JO, Carey RN, Wold S. Criteria for judging precision and accuracy in method development and evaluation. Clin Chem 1974;20:825-33.

7. Westgard JO. A method evaluation decision chart for judging method performance. Clin Lab Science 1995;8:277-83.

Online References

Points of care in using statistics in method comparison studies. Original paper in PDF format.
http://www.westgard.com/essay19.htm

Use and interpretation of common statistical tests in method-comparison studies. Original paper in PDF format.
http://www.westgard.com/method1.htm

Medical Decision Levels.
http://www.westgard.com/decision.htm

Self-Assessment Questions:

○ Linear regression analysis for a glycated hemoglobin test showed that the NEW method = 0.93 (OLD method) + 0.29% (r=0.992). What are the estimates of slope and intercept?

○ Will the estimates of slope and intercept be reliable?

○ Should you use t-test or Bland-Altman instead of ordinary linear regression?

○ Should you use Deming regression or Passing-Bablock regression instead of ordinary linear regression?

19: How can a manufacturer's claims be verified?

In this chapter, Dr. Neill Carey, chairman of the CLSI EP15 committee that drafted guidelines for "User verification of performance for precision and trueness" collaborates with Dr. Westgard to describe the protocol and data analysis recommended for laboratories to verify a manufacturer's claims.

Objectives:

○ Understand the EP15 experimental protocols for precision and trueness.

○ Learn how to perform the EP15 calculations using an Excel spreadsheet.

○ Learn how to perform the "trueness" calculations using paired t-test calculations performed with a spreadsheet.

○ Apply the EP15 guidelines to verify a manufacturer's claims for precision and trueness.

Lesson materials:

○ **MV – EP15 Guidelines for verifying a manufacturer's claims for precision and trueness,**
R. Neill Carey, PhD, and James O. Westgard, PhD

Things to do:

○ Study the materials.

○ Set up the EP15 precision calculations using a spreadsheet.

○ Set up paired t-test calculations using a spreadsheet.

○ Verify your spreadsheet calculations using the EP15 example data set.

Method Validation:
EP15 Guidelines for Verifying a Manufacturer's claims for Precision and Trueness

R. Neill Carey, PhD, and James O. Westgard, PhD

Purpose

Laboratories today are under pressure to manage quality at the lowest possible cost. Even method validation studies raise the issue of cost. What's the minimum study necessary to satisfy the regulatory requirements for verifying a manufacturer's performance claims? That question has been addressed directly in the CLSI EP15 guidelines for "User verification of performance for precision and trueness." [1]

This CLSI document was developed by a subcommittee that represented laboratory users, professionals, manufacturers, and the government. The CLSI process involves peer-review of the recommended guidelines by official vote of its members. Once approved, the guidelines represent "good laboratory practices" that are accepted by the professional community, accreditation and inspection agencies, as well as the government. A laboratory need only reference EP15 to justify the use of these protocols to satisfy the CLIA regulations for validation of new laboratory methods.

According to the EP15 subcommittee, the purpose of this document is as follows:

"The subcommittee had two principal goals during the development of EP15. One was to develop a testing protocol that is simple enough to be applicable in laboratories with a wide variety of sophistication and resources, from the point-of-care or physician's office laboratory to the large clinical laboratory. The second was to develop a protocol that is sufficiently rigorous to provide statistically valid conclusions for verification studies. To meet these two needs, the subcommittee developed a five-day testing protocol and simplified worksheets for all data gathering, statistical calculations, and tests of observed precision and trueness. A computer spreadsheet is provided to simplify and standardize the statistical calculations and tests of observed precision and trueness.

"This document is primarily intended for use when an established method is initially set up in the laboratory. It may also be used to verify method performance after corrective action following a failed proficiency testing event."

Scope and Definition of Terms

EP15 is intended for use by laboratories to verify that a method operates in accordance with the manufacturer's claims. Other CLSI documents provide guidance for manufacturers to make claims for precision (EP5, 2) and trueness (EP9, 3).

EP15 provides protocols and data analysis to verify a manufacturer's claims for repeatability, within-laboratory precision, and trueness. These performance characteristics are defined in the EP15 document as follows:

- **Repeatability (of results of measurements)**: Closeness of agreement between the results of successive measurements of the same measurand carried out under the same conditions of measurement. NOTE: Formerly, the term within-run precision was used.

- **Repeatability conditions**: Conditions where independent test results are obtained with the same method on identical test material in the same laboratory by the same operator using the same equipment within a short interval of time.

- **Within-laboratory precision**: Precision over a defined time and operators, calibration and reagents may vary within the same facility and using the same equipment. NOTE: Formerly, the term total precision was used.

- **Trueness (of measurement)**: Closeness of agreement between the average value obtained from a large series of test results and an accepted reference value. NOTE: The measure of trueness is usually expressed in terms of bias.

EP15 describes 3 protocols: one for precision based on analysis of 3 replicate control samples per day for 5 days; one for trueness based on analysis of 20 patient specimens; and a second for trueness based on the analysis of at least two reference materials having assigned values.

EP15 Precision Protocol

A familiarization period is specified to learn proper operation of the analytic system, including calibration, maintenance procedures, and monitoring procedures (quality control). The manufacturer's recommended QC procedures are to be used to monitor performance during the EP15 testing protocols. Control materials should be selected to have concentrations near medical decision points. The control materials used for claims verification should be selected to have concentrations near medical decision points and close to the concentrations used by the manufacturer in making their precision claims. If possible, they should be the same materials used by the manufacturer in establishing claims, or very similar materials (similar matrix). The testing protocol [1] is as follows:

1. "Analyze one run per day with three replicate samples at each of two concentrations daily for five days.

2. If a run must be rejected because of quality control procedures or operating difficulties, discard the data, and conduct an additional run.

3. Include the daily quality control samples normally used.

4. Samples for the trueness experiment may be tested in the same runs.

5. Calibrate as specified in the manufacturer's instructions for operators. If the manufacturer indicates in its claim that its precision data were generated over multiple calibration cycles, then the operator may choose to recalibrate during the experiment."

EP15 Equations for Precision Calculations:
within run SD (s_r), between-run variance (s_b^2), within laboratory SD (s_l), and effective degrees of freedom (T).

$$s_r = \sqrt{\frac{\sum\limits_{d=1}^{D}\sum\limits_{i=1}^{n}(x_{di} - \overline{x}_d)^2}{D(n-1)}} \qquad \text{Eq. 1}$$

$$s_b^2 = \frac{\sum\limits_{d=1}^{D}(\overline{x}_d - \overline{\overline{x}})^2}{D-1} \qquad \text{Eq. 2}$$

$$s_l = \sqrt{\frac{n-1}{n} \cdot s_r^2 + s_b^2} \qquad \text{Eq. 3}$$

$$T = \frac{((n-1) \cdot s_r^2 + (n \cdot s_b^2))^2}{(\frac{n-1}{D}) \cdot s_r^4 + (\frac{n^2 \cdot (s_b^2)^2}{D-1})} \qquad \text{Eq. 4}$$

Where   D is total number of days,
n is number of replicates per day,
x_{di} is the result of replicate i for day d,
x_d is the average of all results for day d,
x is the average of all results

Data calculations. EP15 provides for estimations of repeatability (s_r) and within-laboratory precision (s_l). The equations are somewhat complicated, as shown on page 225. The calculations involve determining the within-run and between-run variances, then combining the two to get the total variance, which is the basis for calculating the within-laboratory SD. Remember that variance is the square of an SD, therefore the within-laboratory precision is the square root of the total laboratory variance. There is a worksheet in the EP15 document that walks you through these calculations step-by-step, plus there is an example demonstrating all of the calculations.

The EP15 document references a companion spreadsheet for performing these calculations, but CLSI had not released this calculation tool as of early 2008. For this reason, we provide some directions for performing these calculations below. If you have access to a calculation tool for EP15, then these directions are not necessary and you need only understand the results and how they are used to verify a manufacturer's claim.

Calculations using Excel. An example set of data from EP15 is shown in the accompanying figure which also describes how these calculations can be performed using an Excel spreadsheet. For the purpose of the calculations, it is convenient to enter the 3 replicates in a row for each of the 5 days. The mean and SD for each day can then be calculated using the AVERAGE and STDEV functions available in Excel. The last column (G) shows the run variance, obtained by squaring the run SD in the previous column (F).

	A	B	C	D	E	F	G
1	**EP15 Precision**						
2	**Number of replicates**	**3**					
3	**Number of days**	**5**					
4		**Rep. 1**	**Rep. 2**	**Rep. 3**	Run mean	Run SD	Variance
5	**Day 1**	140	140	140	140.000	0.000	0.000
6	**Day 2**	138	139	138	138.333	0.577	0.333
7	**Day 3**	143	144	144	143.667	0.577	0.333
8	**Day 4**	143	143	142	142.667	0.577	0.333
9	**Day 5**	142	143	141	142.000	1.000	1.000
10							
11	*Overall mean*	**AV(E5:E9)**			*141.333*		
12	Within run variance (Vr)	**AV(G5:G9)**			0.400		
13	*Within run SD*	**SQRT(E12)**			*0.632*		
14	Between run SD	**SD(E5:E9)**			2.147		
15	Between run variance (Vb)	**E14*E14**			4.611		
16	Ratio Vr/Vb	**+E12/E15**			0.087		
17	Total variance	**((B2-1)/B2)*E12 + E15**			4.878		
18	*Laboratory SD*	**SQRT(E17)**			*2.209*		
19	**Laboratory CV**	**(E18/E11)*100**			*1.563*		

With the information above, the estimates of repeatability and within-laboratory precision can be calculated by following the steps below:

- Obtain the overall mean by using the Excel AVERAGE function for the data in cells E5 to E9 (141.333 mg/dL for this EP15 glucose example).

- Obtain the average within-run variance by using the AVERAGE function for the data in cells G5 to G9 (0.400 for this example).

- Take the square root of the average within-run variance in E12 using the Excel SQRT function. (0.632, the within-run SD)

- Calculate the between-run SD using the STDEV function for the data in cells E5 to E9. (2.147)

- Square the value determined above to calculate the between-run variance. (4.611)

- Calculate the ratio of within-run and between-run variances by dividing the value in E12 by the value in E15; (0.087)

- Calculate the total variance from the within-run and between-run variances; Note that this is done by multiplying the within-run variance (in cell E12) by a factor $(n-1)/n$ (where n is the number of replicates as entered in cell B2) then adding this to the between-run variance (from cell E15). (4.878)

- Calculate the within-laboratory SD by using the SQRT function on the value above (cell E17). (2.209, which is the within-laboratory SD)

- Calculate the within-laboratory CV from the SD in cell E18 and the mean in cell E11, then multiplying by 100.

This example spreadsheet is set up for the experimental design of 3 replicates for 5 days, but more replicates can be added by inserting columns before Rep.3 (column D) and more days can be added by inserting rows before Day 5 (row 9). The insertions of columns and rows must be done in this way to be sure that the equations for the data calculations remain valid.

Verification of precision claim. EP15 recommends that a "verification value" be calculated to provide an upper limit for the manufacturer's claim for precision. If the laboratory's observed SD is below this verification value, then the manufacturer's claim has been verified. This verification value depends on the number of replicates (n), the number of days (D), the within-run variance (s_r^2) and the between-run variance (s_b^2). The procedure is to calculate a parameter called T, which is the "effective degrees of freedom," lookup a critical value from a chi-square table (C), then calculate the verification value for the manufacturer's claimed precision (s_{claim}), as follows:

$$\text{Verification value} = s_{claim} * C^{1/2}/T^{1/2}$$

The first step is to calculate T according to equation 4 (shown earlier). This calculation is messy and hard to implement in a single cell of an Excel spreadsheet. Because of that, a step-by-step calculation is shown in the Excel spreadsheet on the next page!

	A	B	C	D	E
1	Calculation of T				
2					
3	Number of replicates	3	3	3	3
4	Number of days	5	5	5	5
5	Within run variance Vr	0.40	0.00	4.00	12.00
6	Between run variance Vb	4.61	4.00	4.00	4.00
7	Ratio within/between variance	0.09	0.00	1.00	3.00
8	(n-1)Vr	0.80	0.00	8.00	24.00
9	nVb	13.83	12.00	12.00	12.00
10	Sum above two terms	14.63	12.00	20.00	36.00
11	Square above = Numerator	214.12	144.00	400.00	1296.00
12	(n-1)/D	0.40	0.40	0.40	0.40
13	(n-1/D)VrSQ	0.06	0.00	6.40	57.60
14	nSQ(VbSQ)/(D-1)	47.84	36.00	36.00	36.00
15	Sum above 2 = Denominator	47.90	36.00	42.40	93.60
16	T calc from Num/Denom	4.47	4.00	9.43	13.85

This spreadsheet shows the calculation of T for the EP15 example data set in column B, plus illustrates the range of values that might be obtained for T depending on the relative sizes of the within-run and between-run variances. Note that to simplify the description in the spreadsheet, V_r represents within-run variance (s_r^2) and V_b between-run variance (s_b^2). The EP15 example gives a T-value of 4.47. Note that the range of T can vary from D-1, or 4, to n*D -1, or 14, as shown by the additional calculations in columns C, D, and E. If the within-run variance is small compared to the between-run variance, then T will be low. A low T-value might represent an automated method having very good within-run precision, but having operating variables that cause day-to-day shifts that show up as between-run variance. A high T-value might represent a point-of-care instrument that uses a new disposable cartridge for every test. The within-run variance might be large compared to the between-run variance, in which case T will be high. If the between-run variance is zero, T gives a value of 10. Because T can vary so widely, it will be necessary to go through the "messy" calculation illustrated above.

Once T has been determined a value for C can be found in the table of "Selected percentage points of the chi-square distribution for selection numbers of levels to provide 5% false rejection rate," which can be found at the end of this chapter (p.239). For the EP15 example data, T is 4.47 and 2 levels of controls are assumed. The entry for 4 degrees of freedom (row 4) and 2 levels of controls (column B) is 11.14.

With this information for T and C, a "verification value" can be calculated for the manufacturer's claimed precision (s_{claim}), as follows:

$$\text{Verification value} = s_{claim} * C^{1/2}/T^{1/2}$$

For the EP15 example, the manufacturer's claim for within-laboratory precision is given as 2.00. Given that C is 11.14 and T is 4.47, their square roots are 3.34 and 2.11, resp., giving a verification value of 2*3.34/2.11 or 3.16 mg/dL. The laboratory's estimate for within-laboratory precision is 2.21, which is less than 3.16, meaning that the laboratory's data *verifies* the manufacturer's claim.

While EP15 recommends verifying both repeatability and within-laboratory precision, it will be sufficient to verify only within-laboratory precision because that estimate should be more representative of the performance achieved under a wider range of operating conditions.

EP15 Trueness Protocol using Patient Samples

It is common practice to validate the performance of a new method by analyzing patient samples by both the new method and the method it is replacing. The assumption is that the results by the comparative method represent the correct values and are the basis upon which the manufacturer has made the claim for trueness or bias. That is likely to be true when the new method is an upgrade of the previous method or previous analytic system. If not, then the manufacturer's claim must be carefully examined to be sure that the comparative method in the laboratory and that used by the manufacturer are consistent in performance.

The following testing protocol is recommended:

1. Test 20 samples whose concentrations cover the reportable range of the method;

2. Test fresh samples in the manner typical of routine operation in the laboratory;

3. Measure 5 to 7 samples a day over a 3 to 4 day period on both the test and comparative methods within 4 hours of each other;

4. Evaluate QC to assure stable operating conditions and valid test results;

5. Inspect the comparison data to identify any discrepant results;

6. Calculate the difference between pairs of results and plot the difference versus the comparison value to provide a graphical display of the data;

7. Subject the data to paired t-test calculations to determine the average difference between methods (bias), as well as the standard deviation of the differences;

8. Calculate confidence and/or verification limits to compare the observed bias to the manufacturer's claim.

Data calculations

Paired t-test calculations are supported by many statistical programs. The "paired-data calculator" described earlier in Chapter 7 will perform these calculations and prepare a difference plot of the results (see http://www.westgard.com/mvtools.html).

Calculations using Excel. It is easy to set up these calculations on an Excel spreadsheet, as shown below:

	A	B	C	D	E
1	EP15 Trueness				
2		Test Result	Comp. Result	Yi - Xi	(Yi-Xi-B)
3	1	76	77	-1.00	-3.50
4	2	127	121	6.00	3.50
5	3	256	262	-6.00	-8.50
6	4	303	294	9.00	6.50
7	5	29	25	4.00	1.50
8	6	345	348	-3.00	-5.50
9	7	42	41	1.00	-1.50
10	8	154	154	0.00	-2.50
11	9	398	388	10.00	7.50
12	10	93	92	1.00	-1.50
13	11	240	239	1.00	-1.50
14	12	72	69	3.00	0.50
15	13	312	308	4.00	1.50
16	14	99	101	-2.00	-4.50
17	15	375	375	0.00	-2.50
18	16	168	162	6.00	3.50
19	17	59	54	5.00	2.50
20	18	183	185	-2.00	-4.50
21	19	213	204	9.00	6.50
22	20	436	431	5.00	2.50
23	Sum	3980	3930	50.00	0.00
24		*199.00*	*196.50*	*2.50*	*4.33*
25		*Mean Y*	*Mean X*	*Bias*	*SDdiff*
26		AV(B3:B22)	AV(C3:C22)	AV(D3:D22)	SD(E3:E22)
27	Confidence limits	t-critical	n	upper	lower
28	p=0.01	2.861	20	5.27	-0.27
29	Verification limits	Manuf Claim		upper	lower
30	p=0.01	2.00		4.77	-0.77

Column A can be used for the sample ID number, then the test result is entered in column B and the comparative result in column C. The difference between the test minus comparison results is shown in column D. The averages of the test and comparative results are shown at the bottom of the columns – 199.0 for the test method and 196.5 for the comparative method. The difference between these two averages provides an estimate of bias, which is 2.50 mg/dL. That same estimate can be obtained by calculating the average of the differences in column D. Column E shows the individual differences minus the bias between methods $(Y_i - X_i - B)$. The standard deviation of this column provides the estimate of SD_{diff}, i.e., the standard deviation of the differences.

A confidence interval can be calculated for the observed bias of 2.50 as follows:

$$\textbf{Upper limit} = \textbf{Bias} + \textbf{t}_{crit}\textbf{*SD}_{diff}/(\textbf{N}^{1/2})$$

$$\textbf{Lower limit} = \textbf{Bias} - \textbf{t}_{crit}\textbf{*SD}_{diff}/(\textbf{N}^{1/2})$$

where Bias is 2.50 as calculated for this example, t_{crit} for N-1 or 19 degrees of freedom and p=0.01 is 2.861, as found in the t-table at the end of this chapter (p.240), SD_{diff} has been calculated as 4.33 mg/dL, and N is 20 for the EP15 protocol. The upper limit is 5.27 mg/dL and the lower limit is -0.27, as shown in the spreadsheet.

If the manufacturer's claimed bias is 2.00 mg/dL, verification limits for the manufacturer's claim can be calculated in the same manner, which will give verification limits from 4.77 to -0.77 mg/dL, as shown in the spreadsheet. Given that the observed bias of 2.50 mg/dL falls within the verification limits, these data verify the manufacturer's claim. Note also that the confidence limits overlap the manufacturer's claim, thus they also verify that the data is consistent with the manufacturer's claim.

It is also possible to use the Excel graphical functions to prepare a difference plot of these data, as shown below:

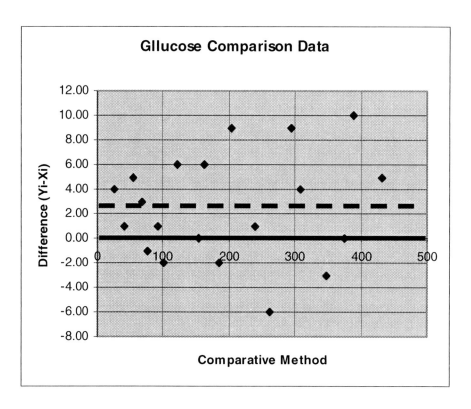

In this graph, the solid line represents "zero" differences and the dashed line represents the observed bias of 2.50 mg/dL.

EP15 Trueness Protocol using Reference Materials

EP15 provides a second approach for verifying the trueness of a method – the analysis of reference materials with assigned values. Such materials must be carefully selected based on their known suitability for analysis by clinical methods and analytic systems. Recommended materials include the following:

○ Certified Reference Materials (CRM) available for some analytes from the US National Institute of Standards and Technology (NIST);

○ Reference materials with assigned values by proficiency testing programs;

○ Manufacturer's materials having assigned values;

○ Materials from external quality assessment (EQA) programs;

○ Materials from third-party vendors that have been assigned values by analyses in several laboratories;

○ Standard materials that can be prepared to known concentrations.

EP15 recommends that at least 2 materials be selected to represent high and low decision concentrations in the reportable range of the method. Materials should be prepared according to the manufacturer's directions, analyzed 2 replicates per run over 3 to 5 runs, then the mean and SD should be calculated, along with confidence limits to aid in verification of the assigned value.

Data Calculations

An example set of data is available in the EP15 document and is shown in the Excel spreadsheet below:

	A	B	C
1	**Reference material with assigned value**		**40.0 mg/dL**
2			
3	Day 1	Replicate 1	37
4		Replicate 2	38
5	Day 2	Replicate 1	39
6		Replicate 2	37
7	Day 3	Replicate 1	38
8		Replicate 2	36
9	Day 4	Replicate 1	39
10		Replicate 2	38
11	Day 5	Replicate 1	38
12		Replicate 2	37
13			
14	**Count**	COUNT(C3:C12)	10
15	**Mean**	AV(C3:C12)	37.70
16	**SD**	SD(C3:C12)	0.95
17	**SE of mean**	C16/SQRT(C14)	0.30
18	**t-critical**		3.25
19	**Upper confidence limit**	C15+C18*C17	38.68
20	**Lower confidence limit**	C15-C18*C17	36.73
21	**SD assigned value**		0.15
22	**Combined std uncertainty**	SQRT(C17^2+C21^2)	0.33
23	**Upper verification limit**	C15+C18*C22	38.79
24	**Lower verification limit**	C15-C18*C22	36.61

The mean and SD are calculated with the Excel AVERAGE and STDEV functions, then the standard error of the mean is calculated to account for the 10 measurements performed. The critical t-value for N-1 degrees of freedom and p=0.010 is 3.25, which can be found in the t-table at the end of this chapter (p.240). The 95% confidence interval is calculated to be 36.7 to 38.7 mg/dL, which does not include the assigned value of 40.0 mg/dL, thus trueness has not been demonstrated by these experimental data.

EP15 recommends accounting for the uncertainty of the assigned value by combining that variance (s_a^2) with the measurement uncertainty from the experiment performed. This is done by adding the two variances, then taking the square root of the combined variance. While the verification limits will be somewhat larger than the confidence limits, the confidence limits will generally be adequate for assessing whether or not the observed performance demonstrates the trueness of the method. In the case of the EP15 example data, the uncertainty in the assigned value was specified as an s_a value of 0.15 mg/dL. When combined with the experimental uncertainty, the resulting SD is 0.33 mg/dL, expanding the standard uncertainty from 0.30 mg/dl to 0.33 mg/dL. The verification limits are therefore only slightly wider than the confidence limits – 36.61 to 38.79 compared to 36.73 to 38.68 – and the interpretation again is that trueness has not been demonstrated by these experimental data.

What's the point?

The EP15 protocol is likely to become the standard of practice in US laboratories for verification of a manufacturer's claims for precision and trueness. For this protocol to provide reliable verification of claims, the calculations must be properly performed. The precision calculations are more complicated than simple replication experiments where one measurement is collected on each material each day. The shorter time period requires replicate measurements each day, which in turn requires that the within-run variance be properly combined with between-run variance to provide a reliable estimate of within-laboratory precision. The trueness protocol with patient samples is more traditional, using paired t-test statistics and a difference plot. However, the trueness protocol using reference samples with assigned values will require some careful thinking and a new understanding of the concept of measurement uncertainty. That will be a step in the direction of understanding the ISO concepts of trueness and uncertainty and the emerging global practices for characterizing the performance of measurement procedures.

References

1. CLSI EP15-A2(e). User Verification of Performance for Precision and Trueness: Approved Guideline – Second Edition. Clinical and Laboratory Standards Institute, Wayne PA, 2005.

2. CLSI EP5-A2. Method Comparison and Bias Estimation using Patient Samples. Clinical and Laboratory Standards Institute, Wayne PA, 2002.

3. CLSI EP9-A2. Evaluation of Precision Performance of Quantitative Measurement Methods. Clinical and Laboratory Standards Institute, Wayne PA, 2004.

Self-Assessment Questions

○ What makes the EP15 protocol attractive for laboratory applications?

○ What are the potential difficulties in implementing EP15?

○ What is "within-laboratory" precision?

○ What is "trueness"?

○ What is the statistical approach recommended in EP15 for estimation of bias?

Selected Percentage Points of the Chi-Square Distribution for Selected Numbers of Levels to Provide 5% False Rejection Rate (Table 1 from EP15-A2(e)).

A	B	C	D
Chi-Square Distribution p=0.05			
df	2 levels	3 levels	4 levels
3	9.35	10.24	10.86
4	11.14	12.09	10.86
5	12.83	13.84	14.54
6	14.45	15.51	16.24
7	16.01	17.12	17.88
8	17.53	18.68	19.48
9	19.02	20.12	21.03
10	20.48	21.71	22.56
11	21.92	23.18	24.06
12	23.34	24.63	25.53
13	24.74	26.06	26.98
14	26.12	27.48	28.42
15	27.49	28.88	29.84
16	28.85	30.27	31.25
17	30.19	31.64	32.64
18	31.53	33.01	34.03
19	32.85	34.36	35.40
20	34.17	35.70	36.76
21	35.48	37.04	38.11
22	36.78	38.37	39.46
23	38.08	39.68	40.79
24	39.36	41.00	42.12
25	40.65	42.30	43.35

Critical Values of t for Selected Probabilities (p) and Degrees of Freedom (df)

A	B	C	D
t-table	Two-sided intervals or tests		
df	p=0.10	p=0.05	p=.0.01
2	2.92	4.30	9.92
3	2.35	3.18	5.84
4	2.13	2.78	4.60
5	2.02	2.57	4.03
6	1.94	2.45	3.71
7	1.90	2.36	3.50
8	1.86	2.31	3.36
9	1.83	2.26	3.25
10	1.81	2.23	3.17
12	1.78	2.18	3.06
14	1.76	2.14	2.98
16	1.75	2.12	2.92
18	1.73	2.10	2.88
20	1.72	2.09	2.84
30	1.70	2.04	2.75
40	1.68	2.02	2.70
60	1.67	2.00	2.66
120	1.66	1.98	2.62
∞	1.64	1.95	2.58

20: How can a manufacturer's claims be evaluated on the Sigma-scale?

The CLIA regulations require that laboratories verify that the observed performance of a method is consistent with the manufacturer's performance claims. In addition, laboratories would be well advised to evaluate the quality of the testing process on the basis of those claims, as well as its acceptability for the intended clinical use. A Sigma-metric can be calculated from a manufacturer's claims for precision (SD, CV) and accuracy (bias, trueness) to provide an objective assessment of quality on the Sigma-scale and to judge the acceptability of the method.

Objectives:

○ Understand the Six Sigma concept.

○ Learn how to calculate a Sigma-metric from estimates of imprecision and bias and a defined quality requirement.

○ Relate that Sigma-metric to the acceptability of performance

Lesson materials:

○ **MV – Translating performance claims into Sigma-metrics,** by James O. Westgard, PhD, and Sten Westgard, MS

Things to do:

○ Study the materials.

○ Review applications of Sigma-metrics on Westgard Web.

Method Validation:

Translating performance claims into Sigma metrics

James O. Westgard, PhD, and Sten Westgard, MS

The Method Decision Chart that was described in chapter 16 provides a graphical tool for judging performance. The operating point represents the precision and bias observed for method, which is then compared with several criteria for judging the acceptability of performance. These different total error criteria describe different levels of quality on the "Sigma-scale," e.g., a method that satisfies the "TE=bias+6s" criterion achieves Six Sigma quality, which is the goal for world class quality, whereas a method that satisfies the "TE=bias+3s" criterion meets the minimum requirement for a production process.

A manufacturer's performance claims for precision and bias can be converted directly into Sigma-metrics to determine the acceptability of a method – to answer the question, "Is this method good enough?"

A terribly short introduction to Six Sigma

In order to understand the relationship between method validation data and Six Sigma, we need to introduce Six Sigma concepts and calculations. This presents a bit of a problem, since this is usually at least a book-length task. In fact, we've written an entire book on the subject: *Six Sigma QC Design and Control* [1]. So all we can provide in this short space, as we near the end of *this* book, is a brief profile of Six Sigma. It should be enough to help you, but bear in mind, there's a lot more depth to Six Sigma than we're going to be able to discuss here.

Six Sigma is one of the popular quality management systems. But the concepts of Six Sigma have been around longer than the trend. Sigma metrics are really the evolution of Total Quality Management with a more quantitative assessment of process per-formance and clearer goals for process improvement.

The principles of Six Sigma hearken back to Motorola's approach to TQM before the turn of the century. Motorola established a goal: **6 Sigmas or standard deviations of process variation should fit within the tolerance limits for the process**, hence the name Six Sigma.

The power of Six Sigma comes from having a universal measure of process performance on the "Sigma scale" to facilitate benchmarking across industries. The Six Sigma methodology can be applied whenever the outcome of a process can be measured. For many processes, poor outcomes can be counted as errors or defects, expressed as defects per million (DPM), then converted to a Sigma-metric using a standard table available in any Six Sigma text [1]. At a time when outcomes are of great interest in healthcare, Six Sigma provides a methodology to describe performance in quantitative terms that are easily understood.

Two approaches for measuring process performance

Six Sigma Quality Management provides a general goal for process performance – six "sigmas" of process variation should fit within the tolerance limits or quality requirement for the product. Given this goal, it is important to measure process performance to determine whether improvement is needed. There are two different methodologies. One is based on counting the defects produced by the process (an outcome measure) and the other based on measuring the variability of the process directly (a predictive measure).

The first methodology (inspect outcomes) is widely applicable in industry and healthcare and depends on counting the number of defects in the output of a process, estimating the defect rate in terms of defects per million (DPM), and then converting DPM to a Sigma-metric using a standard conversion table. Whenever we estimate an error rate, we could use this methodology to convert that error rate to a Sigma-metric. This first methodology is readily applicable to pre-analytic and post-analytic laboratory processes.

The first application of Sigma-metrics to laboratory data was published in 2000 by Nevalainen et al [1]. The authors used data from three individual laboratories, as well as summaries of performance from 300 to 500 laboratories participating in the College of American Pathologist's Q-Probe program. The original paper provides information on sample size and the number of defects or errors, which were then converted into percent errors and defects per million. DPM figures for representative quality indicators from the Q-Probe data are converted to Sigma-metrics in the table below.

Q-Probe Quality Indicator	% Error	DPM	Sigma*
Order accuracy	1.8 %	18,000	3.60
Duplicate test orders	1.52	15,200	3.65
Wristband errors (not banded)	0.65	6,500	4.00
TDM timing errors	24.4	244,000	2.20
Hematology specimen acceptability	0.38	3,800	4.15
Chemistry specimen acceptability	0.30	3,000	4.25
Surgical pathology specimen accessioning	3.4	34,000	3.30
Cytology specimen adequacy	7.32	73,700	2.95
Laboratory proficiency testing	0.9	9,000	3.85
Surg path frozen sect diagnostic discordance	1.7	17,000	3.60
PAP smear rescreening false negatives	2.4	24,000	3.45
Reporting errors	0.0477	477	4.80

*Conversion using table with allowance for 1.5s shift.

The approach of using outcome measures can be applied to virtually any process. The observed error rates for several of these processes are in the 3.0% to 0.3% range, which translates to typical Sigma-metrics of 3 to 4. Even analytical performance, as estimated from proficiency testing data, is only 3.85 Sigma. The best process is "reporting errors" which has a Sigma-metric of 4.80. No process achieves the Six Sigma goal. The overall average of all of these processes is 3.65 Sigma.

For comparison and benchmarking purposes, Nevalainen cited the following figures. Airline baggage handling shows a 0.4% error rate, or 4000 DPM, which is 4.15 Sigma performance. Airline safety (from the normal system of random causes, not assignable causes such as terrorist hijackings) has a very low fatality rate of 0.43 deaths per million passenger miles, which is *better* than the goal of 6-Sigma performance for world class quality. In industry, the minimum acceptable performance for a production process is generally set at 3.0 Sigma. Typical business processes are expected to perform at about 4.0 Sigma. As observed by Nevalainen, typical laboratory processes appear to be at the same level of typical business processes. Just to take a different example, Firestone tire production – the SUV tires that blew out and caused over 2,000 car accidents and over 100 deaths – was near 5-Sigma performance, which is *better* than any of the laboratory processes evaluated by Nevelainen.

Nevalainen's findings were not an aberration; most healthcare processes are not even close to Six Sigma. You may find that statement shocking, but error rates of 1% to 2% are often considered excellent for healthcare processes. Those error rates correspond to 10,000 to 20,000 DPM or process performance of 3.8 to 3.6 Sigma. Actually, we should be striving for error rates of 0.1% (4.6 Sigma) to 0.01% (5.2 Sigma) and ultimately 0.001% (5.8 Sigma).

With laboratory testing, however, it is difficult use the defect counting methodology to determine Six Sigma performance. The problem lies in the definition of a defect for a test result: is a test result a defect when the value is different than its true value? (and how do you determine the true value of a patient specimen if you only test it once?) Or is it a defect only when a test result is outside 2s control limits? Outside some other control limits? Outside the total allowable error? Causes a medical mistake? Causes a fatality? Most laboratories, if using their current tradition of 2s control limits, would determine the wrong count of defects and subsequently calculate a false Sigma-metric. Given this difficulty, we will not use this technique with method validation data.

The second methodology (measure variation) is actually much easier as well as naturally related to method validation data. This technique depends on defining a quality requirement and measuring the variation. Since this is exactly what is done during the studies, all the statistics and data collected during method validation can immediately be used for Sigma metric-calculation.

Quality assessment of analytic processes

It is very easy to assess the performance of analytical testing processes on the Sigma scale. The maximum tolerance limits (quality requirements) can be taken from CLIA proficiency testing criteria or another suitable source; process variation and bias can be estimated from method validation experiments, peer-comparison data, proficiency testing results, or even routine QC data.

Here's what you need from the method validation studies:

- Replication study results (CV)
- Comparison of method study results (slope, y-int, and even r)

Here's what you need from other sources:

- Quality Requirement (CLIA, clinical, biologic or otherwise)
- Medical Decision Levels (to determine critical level)

To calculate the Sigma-metric, you take the quality requirement, subtract the bias observed for your method, and divide by the SD or CV of your method, as shown in this equation:

Method Sigma = (CLIA TE_a – Method bias)/Method CV

The first step for determining the method Sigma is to obtain the estimates of precision and bias at the critical decision level(s) of interest (X_c). Manufacturers typically provide claims for precision at 2 or 3 different concentrations. If one of those concentrations is close to the decision level of interest, then that SD or CV can be used. In some cases, it may be necessary to average the CVs if a decision level is in-between the concentrations of the control materials; other times, it may be appropriate to interpolate between the claimed CVs. It is best to work with CVs because the SDs will change more dramatically with concentration than do the CVs. Also, most CLIA criteria for acceptable performance are given as percentages.

For bias, manufacturers often present their performance claim in the form of a regression line, i.e., $Y_c = a + bX_c$, where X_c represents the decision level of interest, Y_c is the best estimate of the value observed for the new method, and a and b are the y-intercept and slope that have been calculated from the comparison of methods data. Calculate Y_c, then take the difference between Y_c and X_c as your estimate of bias, then divide by X_c and multiply by 100 to give bias as a percentage. Note that all the terms in the Sigma calculation (TE_a, CV, Bias) must be in the same units, either concentration units or percentages.

Example of Sigma-metric Calculation

Let's take a cholesterol example. Here the manufacturer has made a claim for total precision from an experiment where 2 levels of control materials have been analyzed once a day for 30 days:

Claim for total precision
1.9% at 106.7 mg/dL
1.6% at 238.7 mg/dL

For accuracy, the manufacturer has performed a comparison of methods experiment that includes 80 patient specimens that have been analyzed by the new method and the previous generation analytic system (as the comparative method).

Claim for bias
Y = 1.46 + 0.99X

Given that the important decision levels for cholesterol are 200 and 240 mg/dL, let's start with the 240 decision level. To estimate bias at 240 mg/dL, $Y_c = 1.46 + 0.99*(240) = 1.46 + 237.6 = 239.1$. Bias is the difference between 240 and the observed 239.1, or 0.9 mg/dL at 240 mg/dL, which amounts to 0.4% (100*(0.9/240)). Given that the precision at 238.7 mg/dL is 1.6% and that the concentration is so close to the 240 decision level, we can use 1.6% as the estimate. Therefore, Sigma = (10%-0.4%)/1.6%, which is a 6.0 Sigma process.

At the 200 mg/dL decision level, bias is about 0.3% [(200 – 1.46 – 0.99*200)*100/200]. Precision should be between 1.9% and 1.6%, closer to 1.6%, so let's take a value of 1.7% as our estimate. Therefore, Sigma = (10%-0.3%)/1.7% or 5.7 Sigma. In this case, the metrics observed for the two decision levels are almost the same, as might be expected because the decision levels are not too far apart.

Some General Guidance for Calculation of Sigma

1. Find the manufacturer's claims for precision and bias; pay attention to the concentrations where the precision claims are made.

2. Define the decision level(s) of interest to you and your laboratory.

3. Define the quality requirement at the decision level(s) of interest.

4. Use the CV claim that is closest to the decision level of interest, or average the claimed CVs if the decision level is between the control concentrations used by the manufacturer, or interpolate between the manufacturer's claimed CVs if your decision level is closer to one of the manufacturer's bracketing CVs. To be on the safe side, you can also use the highest CV claimed by the manufacturer.

5. Calculate the bias at your decision level(s).

6. Calculate the Sigma-metric.

7. For two or more decision levels, compare the Sigma-metrics to determine which is more critical for patient care.

Scientific judgment will play a big role in choosing the right numbers to be included in the calculations. Manufacturer's usually make claims for within-run and total precision. Use of total precision will usually give a lower Sigma-metric, but will be more representative of the long-term performance in the laboratory. Manufacturers may provide bias claims vs two or more comparative methods. You should select the comparison method most similar to your own method.

Power of Sigma

The Sigma-metric brings together the quality requirement for the test and the precision and bias observed for the method, all in one number. It puts method performance on a single scale, regardless of the test of interest. That scale is a quality scale that has well-established cross-industry benchmarks – 6.0 Sigma is the goal, 3.0 Sigma is the minimum that is acceptable.

You can easily determine the performance that is desirable in a method. For example, given that the CLIA criterion for acceptable performance is 10%, a method needs to have a CV of 1.7% and a bias of 0.0% to achieve 6-Sigma quality [(10-0.0)/6 = 1.7]. One wonders how expert groups such as the National Cholesterol Education Program (NCEP) came up with the guidelines for the maximum allowable CV of 3.0% and the maximum allowable bias of 3.0%. Given the CLIA criterion for acceptable performance, such a cholesterol method would have a Sigma of 2.33 [(10-3)/3]. In any other industry, a process having less than 3.0 Sigma capability would NOT be considered for routine production or routine application. With that one example, you can see how the concepts and principles of Six Sigma can impact our understanding of process performance and change our goals and specifications for analytical methods.

Quality assessment of healthcare processes

Given the universal applicability of the Six Sigma methodology, we can expect demands by the public to know the quality of healthcare processes on the Sigma scale. If we don't make the translation, others will take the reported error rates and convert them to Sigma-metrics. The public will soon have a better understanding of the quality of healthcare!

Would you like to explain to patients why healthcare processes are worse than airline baggage handling? Probably not. We have not properly understood how to assess the quality of our processes and to set goals for process improvement. Six Sigma changes that. Laboratories are fortunate because the concepts can be easily applied and the data required for the calculations is already being collected.

This chapter barely brushes the surface of the concepts, advantages and applications of Six Sigma. Sigma-metrics are a logical extension of method validation and a practical use of the validation data. The calculation is simple and the result powerful.

For much more information, consult *Six Sigma QC Design and Control*, or visit Westgard Web for a list of Six Sigma lessons and applications: http://www.westgard.com/archives.htm

References

1. Westgard JO. Six Sigma Quality Design and Control: Desirable precision and requisite QC for laboratory testing processes. Second Edition. Madison, WI:Westgard QC, Inc., 2007.

2. Nevalainen D, Berte L, Kraft C, Leigh E, Morgan T. Evaluating laboratory performance on quality indicators with the six sigma scale. Arch Pathol Lab Med 2000;124:516-519.

Self-Assessment Questions

○ What is the relationship between the Method Decision Chart and Sigma-metrics?

○ What is the equation for calculating a Sigma-metric?

○ How can you calculate Sigma from a manufacturer's claim?

○ What is Sigma for a cholesterol method where precision is claimed to be 2.0% at a concentration of 200 mg/dL and the accuracy claim is given as the regression equation y=0.96x + 6.0 ?

21: What impact will ISO have on analytical quality management?

This chapter considers an evolving approach to analytical quality management that is being recommended by the International Standards Organization (ISO) in its 15189 guideline for medical laboratories. Following earlier standards for metrological laboratories, ISO places heavy emphasis on trueness and uncertainty. It's important to be aware of this global standard, but also to recognize the strengths and weakness of this approach vs our traditional approach that is based on an "error framework."

Objectives:

O Review the ISO requirements for method validation and verification.

O Become familiar with the ISO concepts of trueness, traceability, and measurement uncertainty.

O Contrast these metrological concepts with the error concepts that have been developed for use in medical laboratories.

O Assess the practical value of the error framework for managing analytical quality in a service laboratory.

O Recognize the impact that ISO will have on US laboratories in the futrue.

Lesson materials:

O **Quality Concepts – Is it better to be uncertain or in error?**

Things to do:

O Study the materials.

O If ISO 18159 is available to you, review sections 5.5 & 5.6

21. Quality Concepts: Is it better to be uncertain than in error?

James O. Westgard, PhD

With the publication in 2003 of ISO 15189, a global quality standard became available that was intended for medical laboratories [1]. Earlier ISO standards had sometimes been used by medical laboratories, even though those standards were intended for general applications, e.g., ISO 9000 series for Quality Management Systems, or for specific applications in metrology laboratories, e.g., ISO 17025 General Requirements for the Competence of Testing and Calibration Laboratories, which emphasized the concepts of trueness and uncertainty following the Guide to the expression of Uncertainty of Measurement [GUM, 2].

With development of 15189, the concepts and terminology that had been applied to testing and calibration laboratories, i.e., metrology laboratories, were applied to medical laboratories. We now live in the world of trueness, accuracy, precision, and measurement uncertainty. New CLSI documents demonstrate that this terminology is being adopted for US laboratories, e.g., EP15-A2 is titled "User Verification of Performance for Precision and Trueness" [3]. In addition, CLSI has a project underway (C51) to produce a document on "Expression of Uncertainty of Measurement in Clinical Laboratory Medicine."

ISO Guidance for Method Validation and Quality Control

ISO 15189 is a "high level" standard that provides general guidance for what should be done, but not many specifics about how to do it. The guidance for method validation and quality control is found in section 5. The references, quotations, and paraphrasing here comes from the 3rd edition that was expected to be published by the end of 2008. Readers are advised to consult that document when it becomes available. The purpose here is to show the future direction of this guidance and assess its implications for analytical quality management.

5.5.1.2 Validation and/or verification of examination procedures. All examination procedures shall be validated to ensure, through the provision of objective evidence that the performance specifications of the procedure relate to the intended use of the examination. For those procedures that have been validated by the method developer (i.e., the manufacturer or author of a published method), the laboratory shall obtain information from the method developer to confirm that the performance specifications of the method are appropriate for its intended use.

> Note 1. This information may also be used, if necessary, to validate the method for an alternative intended use.

> Note 2. The performance specifications of the examination method include: detection limit; quantitation limit; linearity; sensitivity; measurement precision, including measurement repeatability and measurement reproducibility; selectivity/specificity, including interfering substances and robustness.

> Note 3. The laboratory should take into account the desired goal for measurement uncertainty based on the intended use of the examination.

5.5.1.3 Validation of examination procedures. The validation shall be as extensive as is necessary and confirm, through the provision of objective evidence, that the requirements (performance specifications) for the specific intended use of the examination have been fulfilled.

There follows a list of the information that should be recorded:

> identity of measurand, purpose of the examination and goals for performance, principle of the method, performance requirements (see list in Note 2 above), primary sample type, requirement equipment and materials, calibration procedures, step-by-step instructions for performing the examination, QC procedures, interferences, calculations, measurement uncertainty, reference intervals, reportable interval (range), alert/critical values, test interpretation, safety precautions, and potential sources of variation.

For each validation study, the laboratory shall record the following:

> acceptance/rejection criteria, results obtained, control and calibration procedures, data analysis, performance characteristics determined, comparison of results with other methods and other laboratories, factors influencing results, carryover (when applicable), and interferences or non-specificity.

5.5.1.3. Verification of examination procedures. Examination procedures from method developers that are used without modification shall be verified as meeting the needs and requirements of users. The verification procedure shall confirm through provision of objective evidence that specified performance requirements have been fulfilled. The verification shall be as extensive as is necessary to meet the intended use of the examination results. The performance specifications studied during the verification process should be those relevant to the intended use of the examination. The laboratory shall verify the installation of equipment and operation of the examination procedures.

For quantitative methods,

the following attributes shall be verified as meeting the method developer's performance specifications: measurement precision, including reproducibility and repeatability; agreement of patient results with previous or reference procedure; recovery of measurand over the analytical measurement range; carryover from high concentrations, when applicable; interferences or non-specificity; reference intervals or clinical decision points.

For qualitative methods,

the following attributes shall be verified: reproducibility and repeatability for samples above and below the threshold for positive and negative; agreement of patient results; carryover, when applicable; interferences or non-specificity.

5.6.2.1 Quality control programme. The laboratory shall design a quality control programme for each type of examination with the capability to detect error, monitor the performance of examination procedures, and verify the intended quality of results.

5.6.3 Measurement uncertainty. The laboratory shall determine the measurement uncertainty of its measurement procedures for the purpose of interpreting measured values. When calculating the uncertainty of measurement, all uncertainty components which significantly contribute to the measurement uncertainty shall be taken into account using appropriate methods of analysis. The laboratory shall make the measurement uncertainty available to users of the laboratory on request.

5.6.3.1 Calibration of measuring systems. The laboratory shall have a programme for calibrating measuring systems that is designed and performed to ensure that results are traceable to a specified reference material or a higher order, preferably to SI unit or by reference to a natural constant or other stated reference. Where calibrations cannot be made in SI units, the laboratory shall provide confidence in measurements to appropriate measurement standards such as the use of certified reference materials or use of specified methods and/or consensus standards. Reference materials used as metrological traceability trueness controls must be validated to be commutable for the examination procedure for which they will be used.

5.6.4 Verifying the metrological comparability of results. For those examinations performed using different procedures or equipment or at different sites, or all these, there shall be a defined mechanism for comparing the procedures, equipment, and methods used and verifying the metrological comparability of results for patient samples throughout the clinically appropriate intervals. Such verification shall be performed at defined periods of time appropriate to the characteristics of the procedure or equipment.

Intended Use, Validation, and Verification

ISO documents use a standardized nomenclature that may not be entirely familiar to laboratory scientists. For example, the distinction between validation and verification has to do with "intended use." Intended use, a frequent term in the ISO guidance, does NOT explicitly define the quality required for the clinical application of the laboratory test. "Intended use" can be represented by a defined allowable total error, which is the practice in this book. However, it may also be represented by a "clinical decision interval" type of quality requirement (see chapter 2) which is a more direct representation of a clinical quality requirement.

Note also that "intended use" applies to the design of the QC procedure, specifically to "verify the intended quality of results." The "how to" for designing QC on the basis of the quality required for a test and the precision and accuracy observed for a method can be found in our books *Basic Planning for Quality*, *Six Sigma Quality Design and Control*, and *Assuring the Right Quality Right*.

According to ISO 15189, **validation** is defined as *the confirmation, through the provision of objective evidence, that the requirements for a specific intended use or application have been fulfilled.* **Verification**, on the other hand, is defined as *the confirmation, through provision of objective evidence, that specified requirements* *have been fulfilled*. In the context of this book, verification relates to the confirmation of a manufacturer's performance claims, as discussed specifically in chapter 19. Validation relates to the comparison of observed method performance with a defined requirement for quality, which is the primary message of this book, as supported by the Method Decision Chart in chapter 16 and the Sigma-metrics assessment of a manufacturer's claim in chapter 20.

Method performance characteristics

The ISO list of characteristics is very similar to the CLIA list, i.e., reportable range or linearity; precision or repeatability and reproducibility; accuracy or bias or trueness; interference, recovery, and analytical specificity; detection limit or quantitation limit; reference intervals plus clinical decision points or cutoffs. ISO places a stronger emphasis on calibration, particularly the verification of traceability rather that simply demonstrating that the calibrators are consistent with their assigned values (which may or may not be traceable to the true value). The other big difference is ISO's emphasis on measurement uncertainty, a separate performance characteristic that laboratories must determine.

While this book provides detailed guidance on how to define the "intended use" of a test and how to satisfy the ISO requirements for verification and validation of method performance characteristics, the discussion falls short in providing an understanding of trueness and measurement uncertainty. The remainder of this chapter addresses that shortcoming and provides a broader perspective of the directions of global standards and some changes that are likely to be encountered US laboratories in the future.

Trueness and Traceability

First, some basic definitions of ISO/GUM terminology [1,2]:

- **Examination procedure**: set of operations having the objective of determining the value or characteristic of a property; (Note – this is an ISO term that corresponds to method or measurement procedure.)

- **Measurand**: quantity intended to be measured;

- **Accuracy of measurement**: closeness of the agreement between the result of a measurand and a true value of the measurand;

- **Trueness of measurement**: closeness of agreement between the average value obtained from a large series of measurements and a true value;

- **Precision**: closeness of agreement between quantity values obtained by replicate measurements of a quantity, under specified conditions;

A fundamental principle is that "trueness" can be defined only through "traceability." Traceability refers to a framework of reference methods and reference materials that link a test method back to the truth or true value, as shown in the accompanying figure.

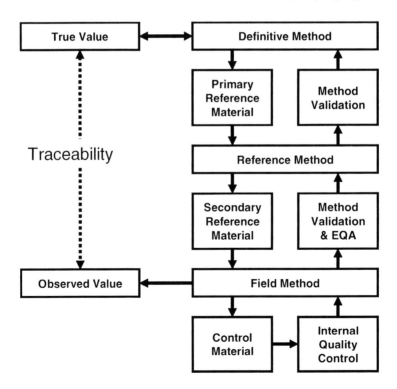

The starting point is a definitive method that can be used to assign values to primary reference materials and also provide a basis of comparison for more practical reference methods. Such reference methods and secondary reference materials become the practical link to the truth for field methods, which are implemented in routine laboratories and monitored by means of internal and external quality control. In this context, internal QC refers to the analysis of control materials by the laboratory and external QC relates to Proficiency Testing or External Quality Assessment programs.

Cholesterol provides a historic example of the development and implementation of a national reference system in the US. A definitive method and certified reference materials were developed by the US National Institute for Standards and Technology (NIST). A series of reference laboratories were established by CDC to support national standardization efforts. Those laboratories utilized an Abell-Kendahl method to provide a reference for comparison of field methods. Manufacturers provided calibrators and field methods that delivered consistent test results in routine laboratory service, where methods were monitored daily using stable QC materials and periodically by external proficiency testing materials.

Based on such a system of reference methods and materials, a "traceable value" can be established for comparison, as shown in the accompanying figure.

"Traceable value" replaces the earlier "true value" which could never be known exactly. Note that ISO/GUM does not actually define the term "traceable value," but assumes that such a value can substitute for the true value. Of course, the traceable value can't be known exactly either and its correctness must be described in terms of "measurement uncertainty" (MU). In this new world of ISO and GUM, accuracy now becomes the error of an individual result, which has certain similarities to total error in that it can be affected by both random and systematic errors, but they are now considered different sources of variance, not different types of errors.

ISO Trueness and Accuracy

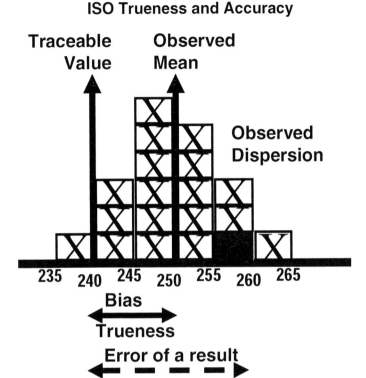

Measurement Uncertainty

To understand measurement uncertainty, it is necessary to become familiar with additional ISO/GUM terminology [1,2], as follows:

- **Uncertainty of measurement**: parameter, associated with the result of a measurement, that characterizes the dispersion of the values that could reasonably be attributed to the measurand;

- **Target measurement uncertainty:** measurement uncertainty formulated as a goal and decided on the basis of a specific intended use of measurement results;

- **Type A uncertainty:** an uncertainty component evaluated from a statistical analysis of series of observations (GUM)

- **Type B uncertainty:** an uncertainty component evaluated by means other than the statistical analysis of observations (GUM)

- **Standard uncertainty:** uncertainty of the results of a measurement expressed as a standard deviation.

- **Combined standard uncertainty:** standard uncertainty of the result of a measurement when that result is obtained from the values of a number of other quantities, equal to the positive square root of a sum of terms, the terms being the variances or covariances of these other quantities weighted according to how the measurement result varies with changes in these quantities.

- **Expanded uncertainty:** quantity defining an interval about the result of a measurement that may be expected to encompass a large fraction of the distribution of values that could reasonably be attributed to the measurand;

  NOTE 1. The fraction may be viewed as the coverage probability or level of confidence of the interval;
  NOTE 2. To associate a specific level of confidence with the interval defined by the expanded uncertainty requires explicit or implicit assumptions regarding the probability distribution characterized by the measurement result and its combined standard uncertainty. The level of confidence that may be attributed to this interval can be known only to the extent to which such assumptions may be justified;
  NOTE 3. Expended uncertainty is termed overall uncertainty in paragraph 5 of Recommendation INC-1 (1980). (GUM)

The concepts and terminology related to uncertainty are illustrated in the next figure. An estimate of uncertainty can be provided in the form of a standard deviation (called the Standard Uncertainty). Estimates from multiple components of a measurement process can be combined by adding the variances of the individual components then taking the square root of the combined variance (called the Combined Standard Uncertainty). Those component variances can be estimated experimentally (called Type A uncertainty) or theoretically (called Type B uncertainty). Finally the uncertainty can be expressed as a confidence interval with a stated coverage factor (an Expanded Uncertainty or Expanded Combined Uncertainty with a coverage factor of 2 for a 95% interval).

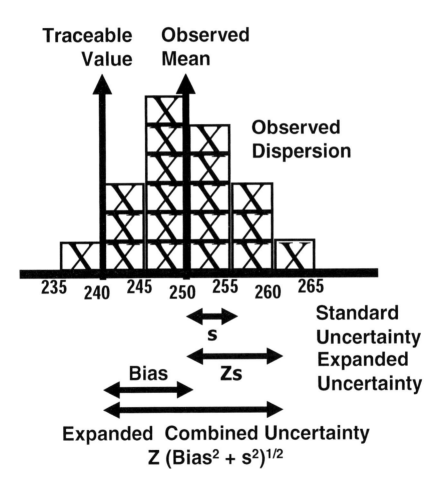

Intended Customers and Applications

It may be helpful to assess the concepts of trueness, accuracy, precision, total error, and measurement uncertainty in the context of the customers who will make use of these concepts. Different customers have different capabilities and/or needs for applying these different concepts. In the laboratory, we have traditionally used an "error framework" to understand the quality of tests and methods. In our changing global workplace, the "uncertainty framework" may not offer any additional utility for assessing, controlling, and managing the quality of laboratory testing processes. Here's why!

In the world of metrology, the intended customers are high level scientists who want to determine the reliability of a value for a certified reference material. In this environment, the intended customers are knowledgeable about the meaning of trueness and measurement uncertainty and are able to incorporate such information into their intended use.

It's quite different in the world of healthcare! Physicians, while highly educated in medical sciences, have little understanding of analytical measurements and their performance characteristics. Laboratory tests appear to provide very exact information, particularly when the results are printed with many significance figures on computer generated reports. Therefore, the laboratory must intervene on behalf of the physician as well as the patient to provide test results that are reliable for the intended clinical use.

Similarly, manufacturers must intervene on behalf of laboratories to provide measurement procedures that provide comparable results. Laboratories depend on manufacturers to provide methods with analytical specificity, proper standardization, and calibrator materials that transfer trueness to the individual laboratory application.

As clinical laboratory scientists, we must recognize what is needed in healthcare testing to manage quality and achieve comparable test results from different laboratories. It is important that these activities and responsibilities be properly focused, in the following ways:

- Trueness must be primarily addressed by manufacturers. If traceability is to be achieved, it will need to be done by manufacturers. Few healthcare laboratories have the time and resources to do this. In the laboratory, the only practical approach is for those assays for which certified reference materials are available and can be used for the traceability of calibration. The practical measure is "bias" which indicates that the systematic concept of accuracy is applied here.

- Accuracy, particularly the residual bias of a measurement procedure after appropriate standardization, correction for bias, and proper calibration in the field, must be claimed by manufacturers and verified by laboratories. The practical estimation of bias makes use of the systematic error concept of accuracy.

- Precision must be claimed by manufacturers and verified by laboratories. Because there may be different experimental conditions for estimation, the manufacturer must describe those conditions as part of the precision claim. The laboratory must then consider those conditions in establishing its own experiment for verification of the claim.

- Total error was intended to be used to rigorously evaluate the effects of measurement performance on the clinical usefulness of test results [4]. Total error should be addressed by both manufacturers and laboratories to establish suitability for "intended use." Unfortunately, US regulations do not require that manufacturers make any claim for quality, though the FDA seems to be encouraging manufacturers to provide an estimate of total error for clearance of waived tests. Nonetheless, laboratories should adopt total error criteria for making their own decisions on the acceptability of methods for their intended applications. As stated in EP21-A [5]:

  "it is recommended that for most cases, if one has knowledge of total analytical error and outliers, then one has sufficient information to judge the acceptability of a diagnostics assay.".

- Measurement uncertainty apparently has some applications intended for laboratory scientists and some intended for the physician user. Laboratory scientists seldom have the mathematical skills of metrologists, thus the recommended GUM methodology is not practical or useful in the laboratory. Physicians seldom have an understanding of measurement variation, thus providing statements of uncertainty is unlikely to aid in the interpretation of test results. In the real world, physicians and patients will probably be surprised to hear that test results are uncertain, disappointed to know they are in doubt, and concerned to hear they may be in error. Physicians are not likely to buy this concept and it will fail in this marketplace. Therefore, measurement uncertainty must be addressed by intermediary customers, primarily the manufacturer and secondarily the laboratory.

Thus, detailed estimates of components of variation are important to manufacturers for improving the trueness and reliability of tests, precision and accuracy are of use to manufacturers when making claims for performance and to laboratory scientists for verifying those claims. Total error is of value to laboratory scientists for judging the acceptability of methods in relation to their intended medical use and possibly to physicians who are interested in understanding the overall quality of laboratory tests. Physicians **do** understand the concept of error!

Utility of the Error Framework in the Real World

From my perspective, total error was a precursor of measurement uncertainty (actually corresponding to an expanded combined uncertainty with a coverage factor of 2). The similarities can be seen in the accompanying figure where the concept of uncertainty is being shown as a "top-down" model that can be compared to the "top-down" model for total error.

Although there are mathematical differences in how systematic errors or biases are added to the observed variance, or imprecision, there is a commonality of purpose which is to describe the range of values that are implied or associated with a single test result. The recommended GUM uncertainty model is a more detailed bottom-up estimate that characterizes each individual component of uncertainty and then combines them to determine

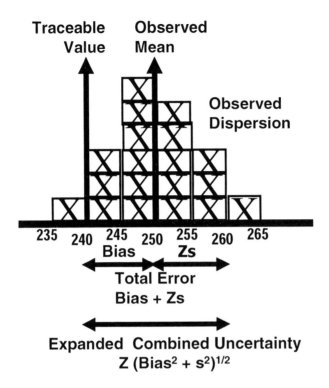

their total effect. That model is impractical in a healthcare laboratory and should instead be aimed at manufacturers and their applications.

Existing guidelines for target or allowable errors. In assessing the reliability of measurement procedures, both manufacturers and laboratories have responsibilities to evaluate and verify measurement performance characteristics, identify sources of errors or variance, and make an assessment of the acceptability of those errors or variances for the intended clinical use of the test. Here's where the error framework has a long history of laboratory applications and many guidelines and sources to assist in the definition of the allowable limits of error. An international consensus conference in 1999 recognized a hierarchy of quality specifications, as follows [6]:

- clinical interpretation criteria, i.e., gray zone between two limits where different diagnostic or treatment decisions are made,

- biologic goals for the maximum allowable imprecision and maximum allowable bias derived from intra-individual and group biologic variation, which have also been combined to provide a biologic total error goal,

- analytical total error criteria for acceptable performance in proficiency testing (PT) and external quality assessment programs (EQA),

- opinions of expert groups (e.g., NCEP), and

- "state of the art" guidelines based on method performance, e.g., as observed in PT and EQA surveys.

Existing method validation protocols. There already exist standard practices, experimental procedures, and data analysis tools to assess the performance of measurement procedures and validate their acceptability for intended use (against quality requirements or target allowable errors). CLSI provides a series of documents that have been developed by technical committees, subject to consensus review and approval, and further modified and revised after experience in the field. These protocols cover precision, trueness or bias from comparison of methods, interference, linear range, detection limits, and reference intervals. They describe data analysis approaches that employ relatively simple statistical techniques and usually include worksheets to guide the data collection and calculations, making the protocols practical in laboratories today.

Compatibility with Six Sigma strategies and metrics. Given a statement of the amount of error that is allowable, there are tools and metrics that fit into today's quality management strategies, particularly Six Sigma Quality Management. Manufacturers have traditionally utilized indices of "process capability" to characterize the performance of processes relative to "tolerance limits" or quality specifications. In the 1990s, those indices were transformed to describe quality on a "Sigma-scale" and to provide benchmarks for quality across industries and across processes [7]. Laboratory applications demonstrate the usefulness of Six Sigma concepts and metrics for assessment of quality of pre-analytic and post-analytic processes [8], characterization of performance and assessment of the acceptability of new measurement procedures [9], and the evaluation of between-laboratory performance from proficiency testing and external quality assessment data [10].

Selection and design of QC procedures. A critical part of managing analytical quality is to perform the proper internal quality control during routine service operation. ISO 15189 [1] identifies the need to do this in section 5.6.1 which emphasizes that QC be designed to "verify the intended quality of test results." Unfortunately, the uncertainty model has not been demonstrated to provide any guidance or tools to fulfill this need. The total error model, on the other hand, can be expanded to provide both analytical and clinical quality-planning models and tools for selecting the right control rules and the right number of control measurements [11-12] on the basis of the quality required for the test and the precision and accuracy observed for the measurement procedure. Thus the total error model has already contributed to the development of a quality-planning process and graphical tools for practical implementation that are already part of a CLSI consensus guideline [13].

Accounting for within-subject biologic variation. In many tests, the within-subject biologic variation may be as large as or even greater than the analytical variation, thus the uncertainty of a test should also account for the patient's own biologic variation. For example, within-subject biologic variation is approximately 6.0% for cholesterol, compared to typical analytical variation of 3.0% or less. Models for goal setting [14] and quality-planning [12] have been developed and are already available. A database of information on within- and between-subject biologic variation, along with goals for precision, bias, and total error, is available for over 300 quantities [15].

Interpretation of patient serial test results. Within-subject biologic variation must be considered in the interpretation of serial test results, which is critical for ongoing treatment of patients. Here's where measurement uncertainty falls short in addressing the intended use and where a solution already exists in the form of the "reference change value," RCV, an uncertainty term defined by Fraser [14] to include both analytical variation and within-subject biologic variation, as follows:

$$RCV = 2^{1/2} * Z * (CV_A^2 + CV_I^2)^{1/2}$$

Where Z corresponds to the "coverage factor" (e.g., 1.96 for 95% or 2.33 for 99%), CV_A represents the imprecision or coefficient of variation for the measurement procedure, and CV_I represent the within-individual biologic variation of the patient.

Communication of results to physicians. Fraser [14] has also developed a practical system for reporting tests results to help physicians interpret changes in test results versus reference limits, as well as significant differences in serial test results, using the following codes on the patient report:

>   higher than reference limit
<   lower than reference limit
\>> higher than reference limit and likely clinically important
<< lower than reference limit and likely clinically important
*   significant change (95% confidence level)
** highly significant change (99% confidence level)

In effect, measurement uncertainty is being reported here without actually providing any numerical values of uncertainty itself. Instead, the estimates of uncertainty are used to determine whether a test result should be flagged as an important deviation from a reference limit or an important change from a previous test result. This application takes into account the physicians' needs for information in a format that can readily be understood and accepted by the customer.

What's the point?

Trueness, total error, and measurement uncertainty have different roles to play and also serve different customers. Trueness and measurement uncertainty should primarily be directed to the manufacturers of medical devices and diagnostic materials, who must be responsible for providing testing processes and materials that are traceable and reliable, as well as providing test results that are comparable from method to method, lab to lab, and country to country.

The error framework, with its total error concept and established approaches for setting quality specifications, is more useful to laboratory scientists who must evaluate method performance, implement QC, and manage the quality of their testing processes to assure achievement of the intended clinical quality of test results. The ISO concepts and principles of quality systems can be applied in the laboratory, as shown by Cooper and Gillions [16], but the management of analytical quality should continue to make use of the error framework and the related approaches and tools that have been developed specifically for the medical laboratory.

Laboratory scientists must assume the responsibility for analytical quality management in order to guarantee the quality of the test results that are produced, rather than just report the uncertainty and expect the physician user and patient consumer to make proper use of the test results. If uncertainty is to be reported, then the system for reporting must be carefully developed by laboratory scientists to aid and support their customers, e.g., Fraser's system for flagging test results based on the reference limits and significant changes in serial test results [14].

The strongest argument for the need to characterize measurement uncertainty will be our failure to properly control laboratory testing to "verify the intended quality of test results," to borrow the phrase from ISO 15189. If we don't manage quality effectively, then we will need to measure the quality being achieved, which can be characterized by measurement uncertainty!

Our world is full of uncertainty, to be sure, but it becomes more manageable in the laboratory when the focus is on analytical errors.

References

1. ISO/FDIS 15189 Medical laboratories – Particular requirements for quality and competence. 2003. International Organization for Standards, Geneva Switz.(Note that a 2ⁿᵈ edition of 15189 was published in 2007 and a 3ʳᵈ edition is expected to be released by the end of 2008.)

2. GUM. Guide to the expression of uncertainty in measurement. ISO, Geneva, 1995.

3. CLSI. EP15-A2. User Verification of Performance for Precision and Trueness. Clinical Laboratory Standards Institute, Wayne, PA, 2005.

4. Westgard JO, Carey RN, Wold S. Criteria for judging precision and accuracy in method development and evaluation. Clin Chem 1974;20:825-833.

5. CLSI EP21-A. Estimation of total analytical error for clinical laboratory methods. Clinical Laboratory Standards Institute, Wayne, PA 2003.

6. Petersen PH, Fraser CG, Kallner A, Kenny D. Strategies to Set Global Analytical Quality Specifications in Laboratory Medicine. Scand J Clin Lab Invest 1999;59(7):475-585.

7. Harry M, Schroeder R. Six Sigma: The Breakthrough Management Strategy Revolutionizing the World's To Corporations. New York:Currency, 2000.

8. Nevalainen D, Berte L, Kraft C, Leigh E, Morgan T. Evaluating laboratory performance on quality indicators with the six sigma scale. Arch Pathol Lab Med 2000;124:516-519.

9. Westgard JO. Six Sigma Quality Design and Control: Desirable precision and requisite QC for laboratory measurement processes. 2ⁿᵈ ed. Madison WI:Westgard QC, 2006.

10. Westgard JO, Westgard SA. The quality of laboratory testing today: An assessment of sigma-metrics for analytical quality using performance data from proficiency testing surveys and the CLIA criteria for acceptable performance. Am J Clin Pathol 2006;125:343-354.

11. Westgard JO. Charts of operational process specifications ("OPSpecs charts") for assessing the precision, accuracy, and quality control needed to satisfy proficiency testing criteria. Clin Chem 1992;38:1226-33.

12. Westgard JO. Internal quality control: planning and implementation strategies. Ann Clin Biochem 2003;40:593-611.

13. CLSI C24-A3. Statistical Quality Control for Quantitative Measurement Procedures: Principles and Definitions; Approved Guideline – Third Edition. Clinical Laboratory Standards Institute, Wayne, PA, 2006.

14. Fraser C. Biological Variation: From Principles to Practice. AACC Press, 2001.

15. Ricos C, Alarez V, Cava F, et al. Current databases on biological variation: pros, cons and progress. Scand J Clin Lab Invest 1999:59:491-500. Note that the 5th edition of this databank (or 2008 update) is available at http://www.westgard.com/biodatabase1.html].

16. Cooper G, Gillions T. Producing Reliable Test Results in the Medical Laboratory: Using a quality system approach and ISO 15189 to assure the quality of laboratory examination procedures. Bio-Rad Laboratories, Quality Systems Division, Irvine CA 2007.

Self-Assessment Questions

○ What is the meaning of the abbreviation ISO?

○ Does "trueness" correspond most closely to precision, accuracy, or total error?

○ Does "uncertainty" correspond most closely to precision, accuracy, or total error?

○ Why is traceability important?

○ What are the advantages of trueness and uncertainty?

○ What are the advantages of the laboratory's traditional error framework?

22. Self-Assessment Answers

Chapter 1: Is quality still an issue in the laboratory?

○ What myths of quality exist in laboratories today?

Many laboratory analysts believe that quality, particularly analytical quality, is no longer an issue because laboratories have implemented quality control procedures, quality assurance plans, and quality improvement projects. We often mistakenly believe that:

- Quality assurance programs assure quality in healthcare.
- Statistical QC controls the quality of laboratory tests.
- Quality can be managed even if the required quality isn't known.
- Quality requirements need to consider only imprecision and inaccuracy.
- Current methods have better imprecision and inaccuracy than needed.
- Analytical quality is a given today.
- No further improvements in analytical quality are needed.
- The government regulates lab tests to make sure quality is acceptable.
- Labs should focus on pre- and post-analytic errors because analytical errors are no longer a problem.

○ What can be done to improve laboratory quality management practices?

Quality must be managed in an objective and quantitative way. This means defining the quality that is needed or desired for each test, performing experimental studies to validate that methods achieve the performance necessary to produce the desired quality, and establishing statistical QC procedures to assure that the desired quality is achieved in daily operation.

Chapter 2. How do you manage quality?

❍ What are the 5 components needed to manage quality?

We often hear about individual parts or components of a quality system, without understanding how they fit together. The total quality management (TQM) framework includes quality laboratory processes (QLP), quality control (QC), quality assessment (QA), quality improvement (QI), and quality planning (QP). These components should function as a cycle or feedback loop to provide continuous improvement of quality.

❍ Where does method validation fit in this TQM framework?

Method validation (MV) should be a standard laboratory process that is employed when implementing a new analytical method. As such, it should be part of QLP – quality laboratory processes. However, it should also be understood that MV is a process that is used as part of quality planning, or QP, to provide the technical assessment of method performance that is necessary for implementing new methods in the laboratory.

❍ Why is method validation important?

Even though manufacturers test their methods extensively, there are many factors or variables that may have changed when the method is operating in an individual laboratory. These factors include such things as different lot number of standards and reagents, changes in instrument or system components, different climate control conditions in the laboratory, different skill levels of the operators, and shipping and storage conditions that may affect reagents and materials. Method validation provides assurance that a new method, with whatever changes have occurred, still operates acceptably under the conditions of use in the laboratory. It's essential for establishing quality laboratory processes.

❍ What drives or guides the quality managment process?

Quality goals, objectives, and requirements are needed to drive the quality management process and guide the implementation and assessment of laboratory testing processes and services.

Chapter 3. What is the purpose of a method validation study?

○ What are the two major types of analytical errors?

The two major types of analytical errors are imprecision and inaccuracy, which may also be described as random and systematic errors, respectively. Random errors can be either positive or negative and their direction is not predictable. Systematic errors are in one direction and are predictable.

○ What is meant by "total error"?

Total error is the net effect of imprecision and inaccuracy on a single measurement or single test result. Because only a single measurement is commonly made when performing a routine laboratory test, that measurement may be in error due to both the imprecision and inaccuracy of the method. Performing replicate measurements can reduce the random error of the test result, but will not reduce the systematic error or inaccuracy.

○ How is total error related to the basic types of errors?

Total error is commonly estimated as the bias (or systematic error) of the method plus a multiple (usually 2, 3 or 4) of the standard deviation (or random error) of the method. For example, using the criterion TE = bias + 3SD, it is expected that a cholesterol test result will be correct within 7.0 mg/dL if the average systematic error or bias for a cholesterol method is 1.0 mg/dL and the SD is 2.0 mg/dL. This assumes that the estimates of bias and SD are appropriate for the concentration level of the specimen of interest.

○ How does your literature report describe the errors of the method?

Most literature studies deal with estimates of precision from replication studies and estimates of accuracy from comparison of methods studies. Reportable range or the range of linear performance is often documented. Detection limit, recovery, interference, and reference intervals are less commonly included. The report may just give a bunch of statistics without any attempt to describe the sizes of errors.

O **What statistics are used in the literature report?**

You will commonly encounter averages (or means), SDs, and CVs for summarizing the data from a replication study. For a comparison of methods experiment, expect to see linear regression or least-squares statistics (slope, y-intercept, and standard deviation about the regression line) and the correlation coefficient, and sometimes also t-test statistics (bias, SD of differences, and t-value). These are the different statistics you need to learn about to be able to interpret the results of method validation studies.

O **How do the report's conclusions relate to the errors of the method?**

The conclusions about the performance of an analytical method are probably the least "standardized" part of a method validation study, even for studies published in reputable journals. They should relate method performance to the "standards of performance" or "quality requirements" of the test.

Chapter 4. What are the regulatory requirements for method validation?

O **What are the test complexity classifications that are used for categorizing the CLIA requirements for method validation?**

The CLIA Final Rule classifies tests as provider-performed microscopy (PPM), waived, and non-waived, where the latter classification includes the moderately complex and highly complex categories from earlier versions of the regulations.

O **What are the method validation requirements for waived tests?**

There are no method validation requirements for waived tests. Laboratories need only to follow the manufacturer's directions.

○ **What are the method validation requirements for non-waived tests approved by the FDA?**

For non-waived tests, the laboratory must verify performance for reportable range, precision, accuracy, and reference intervals.

○ **What are the method validation requirements for non-waived tests *not* approved by the FDA – or – *modified* by the laboratory?**

For non-waived tests not approved by the FDA or modified by the laboratory, analytical specificity (interferences) and analytical sensitivity (detection limit) must also be validated, plus more extensive studies may be required to establish reference intervals.

Chapter 5. How is a method selected?

○ **What are the three types of method characteristics?**

Application characteristics describe conditions that the method must meet if it is to be usable in a laboratory. Methodology characteristics are more technical factors that are related to the performance expected from a method. Performance characteristics are specific measures of performance that are important if the method is to provide acceptable results.

○ **Give three examples for each type of method characteristic.**

Examples of application characteristics would be specimen type, sample size, and cost. If a method doesn't satisfy the necessary conditions, it shouldn't even be considered for use in the laboratory. Examples of methodology characteristics might be the type of standards used (primary vs secondary), the principle of measurement (photometric vs electro-chemical), or the specific chemical reaction chosen (enzymatic vs non-enzymatic). Examples of performance characteristics are reportable range, precision, accuracy, recovery, interference, and detection limit.

○ **Which characteristics are of most interest in method selection?**

Application characteristics must be satisfied in the initial selection of a method. If the method doesn't work on the right type of specimen, doesn't have a small enough sample size, or costs too much, there's no reason to test its performance. Methodology characteristics are also useful in guiding the selection towards a method that is expected to provide the desired performance.

○ **Which characteristics are of most interest in method validation?**

It's the performance characteristics that are actually tested by method validation studies. Precision and accuracy are the fundamental performance characteristics of any method and must always be tested. Other important performance characteristics include reportable range, recovery, interference, and detection limit.

Chapter 6. What experiments are necessary to validate method performance?

○ **What experiment is used to estimate the imprecision of a method?**

A replication experiment is performed by making several measurements, usually a minimum of 20, on a sample that is stable over the time period of interest in the study. Typically a short time period is studied initially, over 1 run or over 1 day, then a longer time period is studied later, over 20 runs and days.

○ **What experiments are used to estimate the inaccuracy of a method?**

The comparison of methods experiment is the one most commonly used to provide an overall estimate of the "bias" or systematic error between the new, or test method, and an established comparison method. Recovery and interference experiments can also be used to test whether a specific material or sample matrix causes systematic errors.

○ Why is the reportable range experiment performed early in a study?

This experiment defines the analytical range over which data may be collected in other experiments. For example, the concentrations of the materials selected for the replication experiment should fall within the useful (reportable) range of the method. Patient specimens in the comparison of methods study should be selected to be in the reportable range of the method.

○ Why are two different replication experiments usually performed?

The quickest information about precision comes from a short-term study, such as a within-run or within-day experiment. If that estimate shows that method performance is not acceptable, there's no reason to go on and perform other studies. If short-term performance is acceptable, then a longer-term study is needed to assess performance under conditions that will more realistically represent what is expected during routine laboratory service.

○ What's the difference between constant and proportional systematic error?

A constant error is one whose size in *concentration* units remains the same even when the actual value of the test result changes. A proportional error is one whose size in *percentage* units remains the same when the actual value of the test result changes. For example, in calibrating a method, an error in the zero setting will usually produce a constant error, whereas an error in the calibration setting will usually produce a proportional error.

○ What experiments are used to estimate constant and proportional errors?

Interference experiments can be used to estimate constant errors (CE) due to specific materials. Recovery studies can be used to estimate proportional errors (PE). Information about constant and proportional errors may also be obtained from a comparison of methods experiment by careful interpretation of the regression statistics (slope is related to PE, y-intercept to CE).

Chapter 7. How are the experimental data analyzed?

O **Which calculations would you use for the data from a replication experiment?**

The mean, SD, and CV are the statistics that are usually calculated. Occasionally, F-values are calculated to compare the observed SDs of different methods.

O **Which calculations would you use with the data from a comparison of methods experiment?**

Linear regression statistics (slope, y-intercept, standard deviation of the points about the regression line) are usually calculated. The correlation coefficient is often included. Other calculations that are sometimes encountered are paired t-test statistics (bias, standard deviation of the differences, t-value).

O **What graphical presentations are associated with different types of data analysis?**

A histogram provides a useful display of the data from a replication study. For the data from a comparison of methods experiment, a comparison plot (test value as the y-coordinate, comparative value as the x-coordinate) is commonly used when regression statistics are being calculated. A difference plot (difference of test minus comparative values as the y-coordinate vs the comparative value as x-coordinate) is often used when t-test statistics are calculated.

O **What are the mean, SD, and CV on the basis of the following set of data [203, 202, 204, 201, 197, 200, 198, 196, 206, 198, 196, 192, 205, 195, 207, 198, 201, 195, 202, 195]?**

The reason for asking this question (and the following one) is to find out if you have access to calculation tools, such as a hand-held calculator, electronic spreadsheet program, or computer statistics program. You can also take advantage of the online calculators available at

http://www.westgard.com/mvtools.html

For this data set (which is also the demonstration data set provided with the online calculators listed above), the mean is 199.55, SD is 4.1861, and CV is 2.0977. In practice, we would round the SD to 4.19 and the CV to 2.10%.

○ **What are the regression slope and intercept and the average bias on the basis of the following set of data [given as pairs where test result is 1st or y-value, comparison result is 2nd or x-value; 218,217; 161,161; 240,244; 193,193; 290,295; 117,118; 118,122; 203,204; 74,74; 114,116; 245,238; 262,260; 203,203; 218,207; 311,304; 362,353; 332,327; 428,423; 163,155; 268,257]?**

This set of data is also the demonstration data for the online "paired-data" calculator available at the addresses listed above. The slope is 1.0226, the y-intercept is –2.6022, the SD of the points about the regression line is 4.754, and the correlation coefficient is 0.9986. In practice, we would usually round the regression statistics to 1.023, –2.60, and 4.75, respectively.

Chapter 8. How are the statistics calculated?

○ **For a cholesterol method validation study, paired t-test analysis of the comparison of methods data gave the following results: bias= 1.74 mg/dL, SD_{diff}=5.90 mg/dL, N=81, and t=2.65. What is the critical t-value at p=0.05? Is the observed bias statistically significant? Is the observed bias clinically significant?**

For N=81, the critical t-value can be found in the table and is approximately 1.99 for P=0.05 (two-sided test of significance, df = N-2). Note that you will often have to interpolate between values given in the tables of critical values. The observed t-value of 2.65 is greater than the critical t-value of 1.99, therefore the observed bias is statistically significant or "real." However, the magnitude of the bias (1.74 mg/dL) might be small enough to be acceptable for clinical use of the method. That's why we don't recommend using a t-test to judge the acceptability of the method's performance. Instead we recommend a graphical technique known as the Method Decision Chart, which is described in chapter 16.

○ **For a cholesterol method validation study, the test method has a standard deviation of 4.0 mg/dL and the comparison method had an SD of 5.0 mg/dL, both estimates based on 21 measurements on the same control material at a concentration approximately 200 mg/dL. What is the calculated F-value? What is the critical F-value? Is the observed difference in precision performance statistically significant? Is the observed difference clinically significant?**

The calculated F-value is 1.56 (25/16). For 20 degrees of freedom (df = N-1) for each method, the critical F-value can be found in the table and is given as 2.12. Because the observed F-value is less than the critical F-value, the difference is not statistically significant. However, the clinical significance of the observed imprecision depends on the size of the method's SD compared to the amount of error allowable. Again, we don't recommend using a test of significance, this time the F-test, to judge the acceptability of a method's performance. The Method Decision Chart will allow you to consider both the precision and accuracy of the method relative to a defined requirement for quality in the form of the total amount of error that is allowable for the test.

○ **To verify a manufacturer's claim for precision, an F-test was calculated to compare the SD of 5.0 observed (N=31) in a replication experiment with the SD of 4.0 (N=31) claimed by the manufacturer. Have you verified the manufacturer's claim?**

The calculated F-value is again 1.56 (25/16). For 30 degrees of freedom (N-1) by both methods, the critical F-value is 1.93. Because the calculated F-value is less than the critical F-value, the data do not show any difference that is statistically significant. In this case, the precision observed in the laboratory is no different from that claimed by the manufacturer, therefore the claim has been verified.

○ **To verify a manufacturer's claim for precision, an F-test was calculated to compare the SD of 5.0 observed in the replication experiment (N=11) with the SD of 3.0 (N=11) claimed by the manufacturer? Have you verified the manufacturer's claim?**

The calculated F-value is 2.78 (25/9). The critical F-value for 10 degrees of freedom (N-1) by both methods is found to be 2.98. Because the calculated F-value is less than the critical F-value, there is no statistically significant difference in the precision observed in the laboratory and that claimed by the manufacturer. Therefore, the data is not inconsistent with the manufacturer's claim and could be said to verify the claim. Note, however, that if a better experiment had been performed with 31 measurements, the critical F-value would be 2.70 and the data would not verify the manufacturer's claim. This is an example that shows having too little data limits your ability to adequately assess method performance against a manufacturer's claim.

○ **To verify a manufacturer's claim for accuracy, a t-test shows a bias of 1.5 mg/dL and t-value of 2.5 for a study of 40 patient samples compared to the same comparative method used by the manufacturer, who claimed there was no bias between the two methods. Have you verified the manufacturer's claim?**

The critical t-value is 2.02 for an N of 40. Because the calculated t-value of 2.50 is greater than the critical t-value of 2.02, the difference is statistically significant or "real." The data does not verify the manufacturer's claim that the bias should be zero between these two methods. However, the size of the bias is small (1.5 mg/dL) and the performance of the method might still be acceptable for clinical purposes. Again, this example illustrates that conclusions about statistical significance and clinical significance might be different. Again, a better approach is to use the Method Decision Chart, rather than depend on tests of statistical significance.

Chapter 9. How is the reportable range of a method determined?

○ **How many levels of materials are generally necessary for validating reportable range?**

The minimum is 4, but 5 or 6 are usually preferable.

○ **What's a practical way of preparing this series of materials?**

A series of 5 materials can be easily prepared from a "low" and a "high" patient pool. Mix 3 parts low with 1 part high, 2 parts low with 2 parts high, and 1 part low with 3 parts high. These 3 mixtures together with the original low and high pools will provide a series of 5 samples.

○ **How many replicate determinations are usually performed?**

A minimum of 2, but 3 or 4 replicates may be preferable.

○ **How are the data analyzed to assess the reportable range?**

In spite of all the statistics that can be calculated, the "gold standard" in assessing reportable range is to plot the observed values or the average of the replicates on the y-axis versus the assigned value for the materials on the x-axis. Draw the best straight line through the data, making sure the line goes through the points at the low end of the range. Visually inspect the graph and determine the linear range where test results will be reliable. Describe this "reportable range" by the low limit (usually zero) and the high limit determined from the graph of your data.

○ **How are the data analyzed to assess linearity?**

Linearity actually isn't the performance characteristic that needs to be validated! It's reportable range that's of interest. However, you can use 1st order or linear regression statistics to fit the data and statistically describe the observed line and the fit of the data. There are more elaborate and more complicated statistical tests for linearity that are available in the literature, but for practical purposes, most people just visually inspect the data and the line of best fit to make a determination of linearity.

Chapter 10. How is the imprecision of a method determined?

○ **How many levels or materials are needed for a replication study?**

A minimum of two different levels or concentrations, and preferably three to provide estimates at low, normal, and elevated levels.

○ **What is the minimum number of measurements generally collected?**

It is commonly accepted that the minimum number of replicate measurements should be 20. More measurements would be better because of the difficulty in obtaining a reliable estimate of the SD even with 20 measurements.

○ **What time period should the final replication experiment cover?**

Most studies adhere to a minimum time period of 20 working days or one calendar month because of the high cost of extending the time period of the study beyond the minimum requirement.

○ **How are the data analyzed to estimate imprecision?**

Calculate the mean, SD, and CVs for each of the materials. Prepare a histogram to document the shape of the distribution.

Chapter 11. How is the inaccuracy or bias of a method determined?

○ **What is the minimum number of specimens that are generally compared?**

A minimum of 40 is generally recommended. However, it may be possible to get by with as few as 20 if the specimens are selected to cover a wide analytical range. If specimens are randomly selected, many of the test values will fall in the reference interval for healthy people and, therefore, more specimens are needed to provide the wide analytical range that is desired for the experiment.

○ How many replicate measurements are generally made?

Duplicates are preferred by both the test and comparative methods. However, it is common to perform only single measurements for methods that have been well-studied by manufacturers or are well-documented by published studies.

○ What time period should the experiment cover?

A minimum of 5 days is recommended for the comparison of method experiments in order to provide representative performance of the methods. A longer period of time is acceptable. Quite often, the data is collected at the same time as the long-term replication study is being carried out, which usually covers a 20 day period.

○ How should the data be calculated when there are two medical decision levels?

It's advantageous to utilize linear regression statistics when there are two or more decision levels of interest. These statistics allow the systematic error to be estimated at any concentration within the analytical range that has been studied.

○ How should the data be plotted if there are two or more medical decision levels?

Use a "comparison plot" where the result by the test method is plotted on the y-axis versus the result by the comparison method on the x-axis.

○ What data calculations might be used if there is only a single decision level?

Linear regression statistics may be used to calculate the systematic error at a single decision level, but it is also possible that t-test statistics will provide a reliable estimate of the systematic error if the mean of the data is near the decision level of interest. If the range of analytical data is narrow, then t-test statistics may be preferable to regression statistics.

○ How can the data be plotted for a single decision level?

Along with the use of t-test statistics, you can use a "difference plot" where the difference of the test result minus the comparison result is plotted on the y-axis versus the comparison result on the x-axis.

Chapter 12: How do you use statistics to estimate analytical errors?

○ The following statistical summary was obtained from a glucose comparison of methods experiment:

a = 5.23 mg/dL, b = 0.999, $s_{y/x}$ = 7.23 mg/dL, bias = 5.13 mg/dL, SD_{diff} = 7.23 mg/dL, t = 8.03, r = 0.996, N = 128.

• What is the proportional systematic error between methods?

There is very little proportional error since the slope is 0.999, which is only 0.001 or 0.1% different from the ideal value of 1.000.

• What is the constant systematic error between methods?

Constant error can be estimated from either the y-intercept or bias, which are 5.23 mg/dL and 5.13 mg/dL, respectively.

• What is the random error between methods?

The random error between methods can be estimated from either $s_{y/x}$ or SD_{diff}, which give identical values of 7.23 mg/dL.

• Why is there such good agreement between the estimates of error by regression and t-test statistics?

Estimates of errors by regression and t-test are in such good agreement because there is virtually no proportional error present.

• Is the systematic error between methods statistically significant or "real"?

Yes, the systematic error is statistically significant or real, as shown by the fact that the calculated t-value of 8.03 is greater than the critical t-value, which is approximately 2.0 when N is 30 or more.

• What does the correlation coefficient tell you?

The high value for the correlation coefficient indicates that a wide range of data has been obtained and the regression estimates of slope and intercept should be reliable.

○ **The following statistical summary was obtained for a urea nitrogen comparison of methods experiment:**

$N = 316$, $a = -0.31$ mg/dL, $s_a = 0.23$ mg/dL, $b = 1.032$, $s_b = 0.009$, $s_{y/x} = 0.97$ mg/dL, $s_x = 13.2$ mg/dL, $r = 0.997$, bias $= 0.40$ mg/dL, $SD_{diff} = 1.08$ mg/dL, $t = 6.58$.

• What is the proportional systematic error between methods?

There is a proportional error of about 3.2%, as revealed by the difference between the observed slope of 1.032 and the ideal value of 1.00.

• What is the constant systematic error between methods?

The best estimate of constant error is given by the y-intercept(-0.31 mg/dL) because, in this case, there is proportional error between the methods, which makes the t-test statistics suspect.

• Why is it better to use the regression statistics to estimate errors rather than using t-test statistics?

Remember that the estimates of errors by t-test statistics are influenced by proportional error, which shows up on both the bias and SD_{diff} terms, even though it isn't either kind of error. Therefore, it is better to estimate the proportional and constant components of systematic error from the slope and y-intercept, respectively.

• What is the 95% confidence interval for the y-intercept?
• Does the y-intercept differ significantly from the ideal value of 0.0?

The 95% confidence interval for the y-intercept can be calculated from the value of the y-intercept (a) ± 2 times the standard deviation of the y-intercept (s_a), where a is –0.31 mg/dL, s_a is 0.23 mg/dL, and $2*s_a$ is 0.46 mg/dL. This means that the 95%

confidence interval for the y-intercept is from – 0.76 mg/dL to + 0.15 mg/dL. Because this confidence interval overlaps the ideal value of 0.0, the y-intercept is not significantly different from the ideal value.

- What is the 95% confidence interval for the slope?
- Does the slope differ significantly from the ideal value of 1.00?

The 95% confidence interval for the slope can be calculated from the value of the slope (b) ± 2 times the standard deviation of the slope (s_b), where b is 1.032, s_b is 0.009, and $2*s_b$ is 0.018. This means that the 95% confidence interval for the slope is from 1.014 to 1.050. Because this range does not overlap the ideal slope of 1.00, the difference between the observed and ideal slope can be said to be statistically significant.

- What does the correlation coefficient tell you?

The high value of the correlation coefficient indicates that a wide range of data has been obtained and that the estimates of slope and intercept should

Chapter 13. How do you test for specific sources of inaccuracy?

○ **What's the difference between a recovery and interference experiment?**

The experiments look similar, but are actually quite different. In a recovery experiment, you add the analyte that the test is measuring. In an interference experiment, you add a different material that potentially will interfere in the measurement of the analyte of interest. The calculations are also quite different because the experiments are used to estimate different kinds of analytical errors. The recovery experiment is used to estimate proportional errors, therefore the results are in percent. The interference experiment is used to estimate constant errors, therefore the results are in concentration units.

○ **What common interferences are usually studied?**

The effects of elevated bilirubin, lipemia, and hemolysis are commonly studied for most methods.

○ **What is the proper way to calculate recovery?**

Because proportional error should be represented as a percentage, the results from the recovery experiment are ratioed to provide a proportion that can then be converted to a percentage. The amount recovered should be divided by the amount added. The amount recovered is the difference between the result for the addition sample and the result for a blank sample. A common mistake is to divide the result of the addition sample by the result for the blank sample, rather than calculating the difference and dividing by the amount added.

Chapter 14. What is the lowest test value that is reliable?

○ **When do you need to perform a detection limit experiment?**

Detection limit should be validated for those tests where low values are critically interpreted. Detection limit is important for forensic drugs in order to document the presence or absence of the drugs. Detection limit is also important for tumor markers that are used to follow the results of treatment.

○ **Which estimate of detection limit will generally give the highest value?**

Limit of Quantitation (LoQ) wil generally give the highest estimate of detection limit. Functional Sensitivity (FS) will give the next-highest estimate. Limit of Blank (LoB) will give the lowest.

○ **Why is the Limit of Detection (LoD) always higher than the Limit of Blank (LoB)?**

Limit of Detection (LoD) is always higher than LoB because it is defined as LoB + $1.65 \cdot s_{spk}$, were s_{spk} is the standard deviation observed for a low-level "spiked" sample.

Chapter 15. How is the reference interval of a method verified?

○ **How many patient specimens are generally needed to *verify* a reference interval?**

According to CLSI guidelines, a minimum of 20 specimens are needed to verify the transfer of a manufacturer's recommended reference interval to the laboratory.

○ **What is the minimum number of patient specimens to *establish* a reference interval?**

CLSI guidelines generally recommend obtaining 120 individuals who represent the group of interest. A minimum of 60 is needed to provide a preliminary estimate.

○ **How can a reference interval be transferred from the comparison method?**

Assuming there have been adequate studies performed in the past to estimate the reference interval(s) for the comparative method, a reference interval for a new method can be calculated from the regression line, or regression statistics, obtained for the data from the comparison of methods experiment.

Chapter 16. How do you judge the performance of a method?

○ **How is a quality requirement incorporated into a Method Decision Chart?**

The scaling of the Method Decision Chart is based on the allowable total error that is defined for the test. The y-axis is scaled from zero to TE_a and the x-axis is scaled from zero to $0.5\ TE_a$.

○ **What's a common source of the quality requirement for a test?**

For US laboratories, the allowable total errors are defined for approximately 80 tests by the CLIA criteria for acceptable performance in proficiency testing surveys. The CLIA criteria are officially published in the Federal Register. For non-US laboratories, there are similar criteria available from other national or professional "external quality assessment" programs.

○ What critical performance parameters are plotted on a Method Decision Chart?

The observed inaccuracy or bias of the method is plotted on the y-axis. The observed imprecision or CV of the method is plotted on the x-axis. It is recommended that the CV from the long-term replication experiment be coupled with the systematic error from the comparison of methods experiment to locate the "operating point" of the method. These results will provide the most demanding assessment of method performance.

○ What are the performance classifications on a Method Decision Chart?

Method performance is classified as unacceptable, poor, marginal, good, excellent, and world class (Six Sigma), depending on the observed location of the operating point. A method with unacceptable performance is so bad that the test quality does not come close to satisfying the quality requirement defined for the test. A method with poor performance might have been considered acceptable prior to the introduction of Six Sigma Quality Management, but Six Sigma established a minimum of 3-sigma performance for any production process. A method with marginal performance is okay when everything is working properly but will usually require extensive efforts to maintain performance under routine operation. A method with excellent performance will be very manageable and controllable. A method with world class performance will require minimal QC to guarantee that the desired quality is achieved in routine operation.

○ **What is your judgment on a calcium method whose observed SD is 0.2 mg/dL and observed bias is 0.1 mg/dL at a decision level of 11.0 mg/dL.**

For calcium, the CLIA allowable total error is 1.0 mg/dL, which at the decision level of 11.0 mg/dL would be approximately 9%. Scale the y-axis of the Method Decision Chart from zero to 9.0%. Scale the x-axis from zero to 4.5%. The observed SD of 0.2 mg/dL at 11.0 mg/dL is equivalent to a CV of 1.8%. The observed bias is equivalent to 0.9%. The operating point (y=0.9%, x=1.8%) shows that method performance is "good."

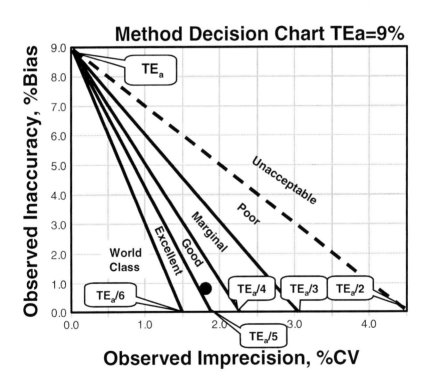

Chapter 17. What's a practical procedure for validating a new method?

○ **What are the minimum experiments needed for your tests?**

The answer, of course, depends on the classification of the tests performed in your laboratory. If only PPM or waived tests are performed, no method validation studies are required. If non-waived tests are performed, you'll generally need to validate reportable range, perform a replication experiment to validate precision, and perform a comparison of methods experiment to validate the accuracy of the method. You can verify the transference of reference intervals by calculation from the comparison of methods results if you have previously performed reference value studies in your own laboratory or by the 20-sample approach to verify the manufacturer's recommended intervals.

○ **What is the minimum number of measurements needed for each experiment?**

Minimum measurements for reportable range are duplicates on a 4 sample or standards series (or 5 materials for CAP). Precision requires 20 measurements over preferable a 20 day period, but shorter protocols may be acceptable for some inspection agencies. Accuracy via comparison of methods should require 20 to 40 patient specimens – 20 if the samples are selected to cover a wide analytical range, 40 if selected more randomly. Transference of reference intervals can be verified with 20 specimens from a defined population subgroup.

○ **What is the best organization of these experiments?**

Perform linearity first, replication and comparison of methods together next, and verify reference interval transference last.

○ **What is the most practical way to make the data calculations?**

This, of course, depends on your personal resources and the resources available at your laboratory. An electronic spreadsheet is often practical because most computers come with some kind of "office suite" that includes a spreadsheet.

Chapter 18: How do you use statistics in the Real World?

○ **Linear regression analysis for a glycated hemoglobin test showed that the NEW method = 0.93 (OLD method) + 0.29% (r=0.992). What are the estimates of slope and intercept?**

It is fairly common to see the regression statistics presented as the equation y = a + b*x, where a is the y-intercept and b is the slope. In this case, y is indicated by the "New method" and x is indicated by the "OLD method." The multiplier of the "Old method" is the slope, which is 0.93. Ideally, it should be 1.00, but the data shows the new method has a proportional error of 7.0% (1.00 – 0.93, which is 0.07 or 7.0% when expressed as a percentage). The y-intercept is 0.29% GHb. Note that the % here is the unit of the GHb measurement.

○ **Will the estimates of slope and intercept be reliable?**

Given that r is greater than 0.99, ordinary linear regression will provide reliable estimates of slope and intercept.

○ **Should you use t-test or Bland-Altman instead of ordinary linear regression?**

It is not necessary to go to t-test or Bland-Altman analysis of the data since ordinary linear regression will be reliable for this data.

○ **Should you use Deming regression or Passing-Bablock regression instead of ordinary linear regression?**

It is not necessary to utilize Deming or Passing-Bablock regression since ordinary linear regression will be reliable for this data.

Chapter 19: How can a manufacturer's claims be verified?

O **What makes the EP15 protocol attractive for laboratory applications?**

EP15 requires minimal data, only 5 days worth or testing for precision, only 20 patient specimens for comparison of methods, and possibly only 2 reference materials analyzed in duplicate for 5 days for trueness. EP15 is intended only to verify a manufacturer's claims, i.e. to demonstrate that the performance observed in a laboratory is consistent with the performance expected (claimed) by the manufacturer.

O **What are the potential difficulties in implementing EP15?**

The calculations are more complicated, particularly those for estimation of precision. The calculations also require estimation of confidence limits or verification limits to demonstrate that laboratory performance is consistent with the claims of the manufacturer.

O **What is "within-laboratory" precision?**

This is a new term, consistent with terminology from the International Organization for Standardization (ISO), for total or day-to-day precision.

O **What is "trueness"?**

This is the new term, again from ISO, for accuracy, which is estimated by the calculation of "bias."

O **What is the statistical approach recommended in EP15 for estimation of bias?**

Paired t-test statistics, along with a difference plot for graphical display of the patient data.

Chapter 20: How can a manufacturer's claims be evaluated on the Sigma-scale?

○ What is the relationship between the Method Decision Chart and Sigma-metrics?

The criteria on the Method Decision Chart correspond to performance on the Sigma-scale, e.g., TE=bias+6s corresponds to 6-Sigma performance, TE=bias+5s corresponds to 5-Sigma performance, etc. You can use a graphical tool to help judge the acceptability of performance, or you can calculate a Sigma-metric.

○ What is the equation for calculating a Sigma-metric?

$Sigma = (TE_a - bias)/CV$, where TE_a is commonly taken as the allowable total error given by the CLIA criteria for acceptable performance in proficiency testing, bias is the accuracy (systematic error, trueness) determined by a comparison of methods experiment, and CV is the precision determined from a replication experiment. All of these quantities must be in the same units, either % or concentration units.

○ How can you calculate Sigma from a manufacturer's claim?

Manufacturers must make claims for precision and accuracy. The precision claim is often presented as the observed SDs or CVs for 2 or more different control materials having different concentrations. The accuracy claim is often presented by the regression statistics obtained from the comparison of methods data. You have to properly interpret the available statistics to come up with the estimate of precision and bias, then plug those numbers into the sigma equation. This requires definition of the "medical decision level(s)" or concentration(s) critical for the clinical use and interpretation of the test result in order to make appropriate estimates of precision and bias from the manufacturer's claims

○ **What is Sigma for a cholesterol method where precision is claimed to be 2.0% at a concentration of 200 mg/dL and the accuracy claim is given as the regression equation y = 0.96x + 6.0?**

Given the CLIA TE_a of 10% and a decision level of 200 mg/dL, the CV of 2.0% represents the performance at the critical concentration. Bias at 200 mg/dL is estimated as 1.0% (Y_c=198 corresponding to an X_c of 200, or a bias of 2.0 mg/dL, which is 1.0% at a concentration of 200 mg/dL). Sigma = (10 – 1) / 2 or 4.5.

Chapter 21: What impact will ISO have on method validation?

○ **What is the meaning of the abbreviation ISO?**

International Organization for Standardization, which sets global standards for the quality management, including a specific document 15189 for medical laboratories.

○ **Does "trueness" correspond to precision, accuracy, or total error?**

Accuracy, which is estimated as bias, or the average difference between observed measurements and the true or traceable value.

○ **Does "uncertainty" correspond to precision, accuracy, or total error?**

Total error represents the maximum expected error from a method of measurement; likewise, uncertainty accounts for the overall expected variation. The two characteristics are calculated in different ways, but both attempt to characterize the quality of a measurement or test result.

○ **Why is traceability important?**

Traceability is the link to the truth or the relationship of an observed value and the true value. Traceability depends on a system of reference methods and reference materials that link field methods back to the truth.

○ **What are the advantages of trueness and uncertainty?**

These terms represent the global standard language for describing the performance of measurement procedures. They are based on concepts and procedures from the field of metrology, i.e., the science of measurements. As such, they represent accepted concepts and terminology that are to be adopted in all fields of measurement and are now being adopted globally in medical laboratories. Trueness and uncertainty provide measures of the quality being achieved by laboratory testing processes.

○ **What are the advantages of the laboratory's traditional error framework?**

Practicality! Errors are meaningful measures of the quality of laboratory tests and measurement processes. People understand that errors need to be carefully monitored and controlled in order to provide test results with the appropriate quality. Many tools exist for measuring, monitoring, controlling, validating, and evaluating the quality of laboratory tests and testing processes.

Answers to Problem Set – Cholesterol Method Validation Data

Linearity experiment

Average values to be plotted on the y-axis versus assigned or bottle values on the x-axis are as follows: 49.50 mg/dL vs 50 mg/dL; 99.75 vs 100; 153.25 vs 150; 195.00 vs 200; 250.75 vs 250; 308.50 vs 300; 341.75 vs 350; 389.75 vs 400. Drawing a straight line through these data points shows good linearity throughout the range. The "fall-off" at 400 mg/dL is 10.25 mg/dL, which is small compared to the allowable error of 10% (the CLIA PT criterion for acceptable performance), which is an allowable error of 40 mg/dL at the high end. Conclude reportable range has been validated as 0 to 400 mg/dL.

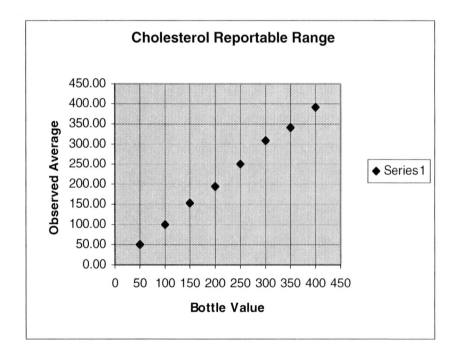

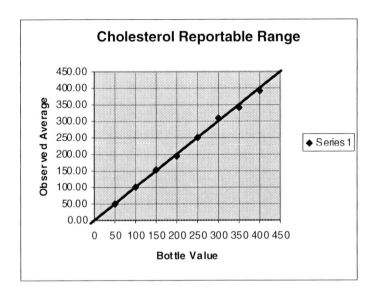

Replication experiment

Data for Control A gives a mean of 199.20 mg/dL, SD of 5.84 mg/dL, and CV of 2.93%. Control B shows a mean of 239.65 mg/dL, SD of 5.61 mg/dL, and CV of 2.34%.

Recovery experiment

The amount of standard added is 50.0 mg/dL (10-fold dilution of a 500 mg/dL standard). For the 6 recovery samples, the average baseline result, average spiked result, difference, and % recovery are as follows:

Base	Spiked	Difference	Added	Recov.
149.75	200.50	50.75	50.0	101.5%
182.75	228.50	45.75	50.0	91.5%
201.75	253.25	51.50	50.0	103.0%
189.00	240.50	51.50	50.0	103.0%
160.50	207.75	47.25	50.0	94.5%
190.25	242.25	52.00	50.0	104.0%

The average recovery is 99.58%, which is very close to the ideal recovery of 100.0%. Conclude there is little if any proportional systematic error observed for this method.

Interference experiment

The effect of bilirubin on method performance can be seen by calculating the difference between the average baseline samples and the average spiked samples.

Base	Spiked	Difference
214.25	225.50	11.25 mg/dL
220.25	234.75	14.50
295.00	302.00	7.00
171.25	183.50	12.25
251.75	260.00	8.25
225.50	236.00	10.50

The average interference is 10.63 mg/dL when the specimen has a bilirubin level of 10 mg/dL. Conclude that an elevated bilirubin is a problem with this method of measuring cholesterol.

Comparison of methods experiment

The original 40 pairs of data show there is 1 pair for which there likely was an error made in recording the results. Sample #8 shows tabulated results of 197 for the comparative method and 275 for the test method. Including this pair of results was a dirty trick to teach you the importance of inspecting the data carefully as soon as the analytical results are available.

If this discrepant point is included in the statistical analysis of the data, regression statistics give a slope of 0.941, y-intercept of 3.25 mg/dL, SD of 15.3 mg/dL for the residuals or points about the regression line, and a correlation coefficient of 0.945. Paired t-test statistics give a bias of –9.73 mg/dL at a mean of 211.5 mg/dL, a SD of differences of 15.4 mg/dL, and a t-value of 4.00.

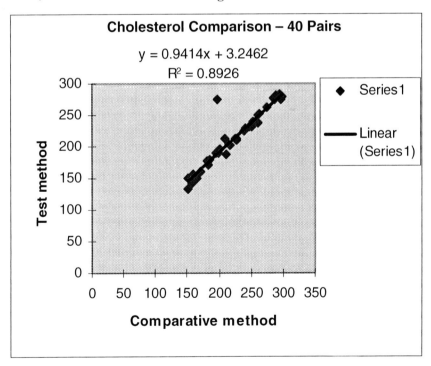

If this discrepant point is removed from the data set and the remaining 39 pairs of results are analyzed, regression statistics gives a slope of 0.967, a y-intercept of –4.70 mg/dL, an SD of 5.73 mg/dL for the points about the regression line, and a correlation coefficient of 0.992. Paired t-test statistics gives a bias of –12.0 mg/dL at a mean of 209.9 mg/dL, an SD of differences of 5.86 mg/dL, and a t-value of 12.8. The discrepant point provides greatest influence on the SD terms and the correlation coefficient because it is in the middle of the analytical range of the data. If a similar discrepancy were located near the upper or lower end of the analytical range, the slope and intercept would be much more greatly affected.

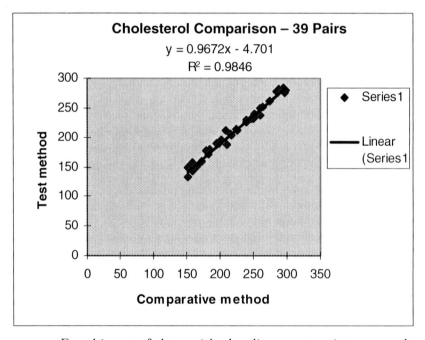

For this set of data with the discrepant point removed, regression statistics are the best choice of analyzing the data. The high correlation coefficient indicates the analytical range of the data is sufficiently wide and the regression coefficients (slope and y-intercept) should be reliable.

At a decision level concentration of 200 mg/dL (which would critical for interpretation of a cholesterol test), the systematic error can be calculated from the regression line, as follows: $Y_c = a + bX_c$, where X_c is 200 mg/dL, a is –4.70 mg/dL, and b is 0.967 The corresponding Y_c value would be 188.7 mg/dL, which indicates a systematic error of 11.3 mg/dL or 5.65%.

Detection Limit Problem Set

Limit of Blank (LoB) can be calculated from the "0" standard as $1.65*0.26 = 0.43$. Limit of Detection (LoD) can be calculated from the SD of the "2" standard plus the previously calculated LoB, i.e. LoB $+ 1.65 * 0.56 = 1.37$. Functional sensitivity is more easily calculated than the Limit of Quantitation (LoQ) The CV of the "6" standard is very close to 20%, the FS is approximately 6.0. LoQ will be higher, but it is difficult to estimate from these data.

	Std 0	Std 2	Std 4	Std 6	Std 8
	-0.23	2.84	5.51	6.46	6.92
	0.12	2.26	5.07	5.14	6.29
	-0.40	1.25	3.15	3.78	8.67
	0.13	3.52	2.72	7.28	7.86
	0.05	1.95	3.67	6.20	5.24
	0.18	2.71	5.35	5.00	7.38
	-0.41	3.07	5.22	5.54	7.41
	0.20	2.47	4.46	6.44	6.06
	-0.32	1.95	2.55	6.71	7.53
	-0.08	1.94	3.61	7.17	10.11
	-0.41	1.93	3.79	4.92	8.70
	-0.39	2.45	3.21	4.40	6.37
	-0.32	2.38	3.42	6.11	7.54
	-0.37	1.37	4.73	7.51	9.30
	-0.17	1.58	4.07	6.38	8.10
	0.38	2.46	3.47	5.55	7.87
	-0.31	2.55	3.28	8.19	8.20
	-0.41	2.57	5.67	8.48	7.99
	0.10	2.27	4.99	5.45	9.38
	-0.30	1.57	4.42	7.61	8.22
	Std 0	**Std 2**	**Std 4**	**Std 6**	**Std 8**
mean	**-0.15**	**2.25**	**4.12**	**6.22**	**7.76**
SD	**0.26**	**0.57**	**0.97**	**1.26**	**1.20**
CV	**-173.50**	**25.44**	**23.46**	**20.28**	**15.44**

Judgment on method performance

A Method Decision Chart can be constructed using this data for a 10% analytical quality requirement, which is given by CLIA as the allowable total error for a cholesterol test. The operating point is represented by an x-coordinate of 2.93% which comes from the data for Control A (whose mean is close to 200 mg/dL) from the replication experiment. The y-coordinate is 5.65% on the basis of the systematic error observed at a level of 200 mg/dL from the comparison of methods data. The Method Decision Chart classifies this method as having unacceptable performance, therefore, you should not consider using this method for routine testing in your laboratory.

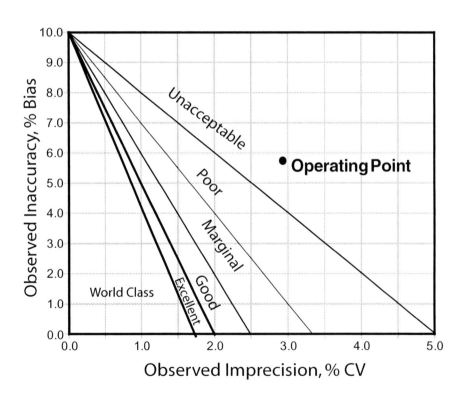

Appendix 1: Quality Requirements

Fundamental to method validation is knowing the performance that needs to be acheived by the method. A quality requirement must be defined if the method validation is to be rational and objective.

Analytical quality requirements

Analytical quality requirements have been defined by the CLIA-88 proficiency testing (PT) criteria for acceptable performance [Federal Register February 28, 1992;57(40):7002-7186]. These criteria are presented in three different ways:

- as absolute concentration limits, e.g., target value ± 1 mg/dL for calcium;

- as a percentage, e.g., target value ± 10% for albumin, cholesterol, and total protein;

- as the distribution of a survey group, e.g., target value ± 3 standard deviations (SD) for thyroid stimulating hormone.

In a few cases, two sets of limits are given, e.g., the glucose requirement is given as the target value ± 6 mg/dL or ± 10% (whichever is greater).

The CLIA PT criteria specify the total errors that are allowable. The total error format is implicit because the CLIA-88 rules specify that only a single test is to be performed for each PT specimen. Under such conditions, the observed analytical error will be the total error due to both inaccuracy and imprecision.

Following is a list of the CLIA proficiency testing criteria for the currently regulated analytes, based on the February 28, 1992, Federal Register.

Note: For the most up-to-date news and information on CLIA, check **http://www.westgard.com/clia.htm**

Routine Chemistry

Test or Analyte	Acceptable Performance
Alanine aminotransferase (ALT)	Target value ± 20%
Albumin	Target value ± 10%
Alkaline phosphatase	Target value ± 30%
Amylase	Target value ± 30%
Aspartate aminotransferase (AST)	Target value ± 20%
Bilirubin, total	Target value ± 0.4 mg/dL or ± 20% (greater)
Blood gas pO_2	Target value ± 3 SD
Blood gas pCO_2	Target value ± 5 mm Hg or ± 8% (greater)
Blood gas pH	Target value ± 0.04
Calcium, total	Target value ± 1.0 mg/dL
Chloride	Target value ± 5%
Cholesterol, total	Target value ± 10%
Cholesterol, high density lipoprotein	Target value ± 30%
Creatine kinase	Target value ± 30%
Creatine kinase isoenzymes	MB elevated (present or absent) or Target value ± 3 SD
Creatinine	Target value ± 0.3 mg/dL or ± 15% (greater)
Glucose	Target value ± 6 mg/dL or ± 10% (greater)
Iron, total	Target value ± 20%
Lactate dehydrogenase (LDH)	Target value ± 20%
LDH isoenzymes	LDH1/LDH2 (+ or -) or Target value ± 30%
Magnesium	Target value ± 25%
Potassium	Target value ± 0.5 mmol/L
Sodium	Target value ± 4 mmol/L
Total protein	Target value ± 10%
Triglycerides	Target value ± 25%
Urea Nitrogen	Target value ± 2 mg/dL or ± 9% (greater)
Uric acid	Target value ± 17%

Toxicology

Test or Analyte	Acceptable Performance
Alcohol, blood	Target value ± 25%
Blood lead	Target value ± 10% or ± 4 mcg/dL (greater)
Carbamazepine	Target value ± 25%
Digoxin	Target value ± 20% or 0.2 ng/mL (greater)
Ethosuximide	Target value ± 20%
Gentamicin	Target value ± 25%
Lithium	Target value ± 0.3 mmol/L or ± 20% (greater)
Phenobarbital	Target value ± 20%
Phenytoin	Target value ± 25%
Primidone	Target value ± 25%
Procainamide (and metabolite)	Target value ± 25%
Quinidine	Target value ± 25%
Theophylline	Target value ± 25%
Tobramycin	Target value ± 25%
Valproic acid	Target value ± 25%

Hematology

Test or Analyte	Acceptable Performance
Cell identification	90% or greater consensus on identification
White cell differential	Target ± 3 SD based on percentage of different types of white cells
Erythrocyte count	Target ± 6%
Hematocrit	Target ± 6%
Hemoglobin	Target ± 7%
Leukocyte count	Target ± 15%
Platelet count	Target ± 25%
Fibrinogen	Target ± 20%
Partial thromboplastin time	Target ± 15%
Prothrombin time	Target ± 15%

Endocrinology

Test or Analyte	Acceptable Performance
Cortisol	Target value ± 25%
Free thyroxine	Target value ± 3 SD
Human chorionic gonadotropin	Target value ± 3 SD or (positive or negative)
T_3 uptake	Target value ± 3 SD by method
Triiodothyronine	Target value ± 3 SD
Thyroid stimulating hormone	Target value ± 3 SD
Thyroxine	Target value ± 20% or 1.0 mcg/dL (greater)

General immunology

Test or Analyte	Acceptable Performance
Alpha-1 antitrypsin	Target value ± 3 SD
Alpha-fetoprotein	Target value ± 3 SD
Antinuclear antibody	Target value ± 2 dilution or (pos. or neg.)
Antistreptolysin O	Target value ± 2 dilution or (pos. or neg.)
Anti-Human Immunodeficiency virus	Reactive or nonreactive
Complement C3	Target value ± 3 SD
Complement C4	Target value ± 3 SD
Hepatitis (HBsAg, anti-HBc, HBeAg)	Reactive (positive) or nonreactive (negative)
IgA	Target value ± 3 SD
IgE	Target value ± 3 SD
IgG	Target value ± 25%
IgM	Target value ± 3 SD
Infectious mononucleosis	Target value ± 2 dilution or (pos. or neg.)
Rheumatoid factor	Target value ± 2 dilution or (pos. or neg.)
Rubella	Target value ± 2 dilution or (pos. or neg.)

Index

A

acceptability of method   11, 30, 33, 62,
    66, 68, 93, 119, 129, 130, 158,
    162, 188, 214, 215, 216, 217, 218
acceptable control limits   45
acceptable performance   23
acceptable range   189
accuracy   10, 42, 46, 48, 54, 56, 57,
    62, 66, 125, 156, 198, 214, 259,
    257, 262, 263, 267
accuracy of measurement
  ISO definition   257
administrative validation   9
allowable bias   188
allowable imprecision   79, 191
allowable inaccuracy   79, 191
allowable SD   188
allowable total error (TE$_a$)   19- 22, 56, 62,
    76, 107, 109, 110, 119, 131, 132,
    150, 151, 163, 170, 188, 189,
    194, 201, 203, 214, 263-266, 269
    see also total allowable error
Analysis of Variance (ANOVA)   120
analytical errors   11, 29, 30, 31, 64,
    84, 98, 119, 138
    definitions   31– 33
analytical measurement range (AMR)   104-
    105
analytical operating specifications   21
analytical outcome criteria   21
analytical quality   6, 7, 16, 17
analytical quality requirements   23, 131,
    163, 188
analytical range   103, 213
analytical run   65
analytical sensitivity   42, 46, 48, 54,
    168, 199
analytical specificity   42, 46, 48, 54, 199
application characteristics   54-57, 203, 214
appropriate QC procedures   22
arbitrary control   22
assigned target values   35
assigned values   107
average difference between methods   141

B

b, see slope
Barnett   18
bathroom scale   63
best line of fit   30, 129
between-run SD   227
between-run variance   226, 227, 228, 229
between-subject biologic variation   271
bias   32, 56, 63, 78, 90, 93, 130,
    131, 141, 143, 146, 158, 163,
    173, 188, 190, 191, 192, 201,
    206, 214, 215, 231, 233, 246,
    247, 263, 264, 265, 266
bilirubin   56, 156, 166, 199
biologic detection limit   168
biologic goals   23, 267
biological variation   7
Bland-Altman plot   213, 217
blank sample   200

C

calculated biologic allowable total errors   23
calculated t-value   141
calibration   40, 43, 54, 56, 63, 66, 67,
    159, 203, 215, 254-255, 256, 263
        definition   104
        manufacturer directions   102
        material   4, 110
        multi-point   102
        set-point   103
        two-point   102
        zero point   103
calibration verification   40, 44, 102, 109,
        data analysis   110
        definition   104
CAP Today   57

Certified Reference Materials   133, 235,
    258
chi-square distribution   230
CLIA, CLIA criteria for acceptability, etc.
    23, 24, 37, 67, 76, 109, 119, 131,
    158, 162, 180, 189, 190, 198,
    199, 200, 246
CLIA Final Rule   8, 33, 38, 39, 41, 48,
    67, 103, 109, 180, 198, 222, 241,
    256

Clinical Chemistry journal   201
Clinical Laboratory Improvement Amendments
   see CLIA
Clinical Laboratory Standards Institute
      see CSLSI
clinical outcome criteria, pathways, practice
   guidelines   21-22
clinical significance   149, 150, 151
clinical validation   10
clinically reportable range (CRR)   104-105
closeness of agreement   223
CLSI   67, 106, 120, 157, 168, 172,
   178, 182, 222, 266
CMS   8, 25, 38, 41, 45
coefficient of variation (CV)   31, 77, 84-85,
   114, 118, 120, 122, 190, 201, 268
      definition   85
COLA   25, 38
College of American Pathologists (CAP)
   19, 25, 37, 38, 47, 48
combined standard uncertainty   261
   ISO definition   260
comparability of test results   262
comparative method   64, 68, 94, 96,
   124, 125, 157, 183, 230, 233, 247
comparison of methods study   29, 32, 42,
   43, 64, 66, 67, 68, 73, 75, 77,
   78, 90, 92, 96, 124, 129, 182,
   183, 190, 199, 201-203, 206, 214,
   217, 246, 247, 266
   appropriate statistics   128–130
   comparative method   124–125
   criteria for acceptable performance   130–
   131
   data analysis   127
   factors to consider   124– 134
   future directions   133
   graphing the data   127
   number of patient specimens   125
   recommended minimum studies   132
   single vs duplicate measurements   125
   time period   126
   verification of manufacturer's claim   131–
   132
   worksheets 204, 208, 210
comparison plot   64, 74, 77, 78, 128,
   142, 150, 202, 204, 212, 215, 216
complexity   41
confidence interval   86-89, 132, 233

constant error   31, 32, 128, 142, 143,
   144, 146, 148, 154,
constant systematic error   63, 64, 65,
   77, 129, 139, 163, 199, 201, 214,
Continuous Quality Improvement (CQI)   7,
   17, 18
control materies   64, 116, 117, 120,
   122, 201, 224
control rules   11, 205
control solutions   116
control values   45
correlation coefficient (r)   29, 30, 77, 78,
   84, 99, 129, 138, 141, 144, 145,
   146, 147, 150, 202, 216
      definition   99
cost-per-test   54
covariances   260
critical concentration level   148
critical decision level   202, 246, 248
      see also medical decision level
critical t-value   149, 237
critical-size error   22
customer focus   17
CV see coefficient of variation

D

data analysis tool kit   72, 138, 200
data-analysis strategy   150
decision calculator   74, 79
decision criteria   11
decision intervals   22
decision levels   215
decision on method performance   188–196
defects per million (DPM)   243
definitive method   124
degrees of freedom (df)   85, 88, 92, 94,
   98, 120, 230, 233, 237
Deming regression   78, 149, 151, 212,
   217
detection limit study   34, 43, 54, 62, 66,
   68, 168, 199, 200, 202, 266
   blank sample   170
   blank solution
      definition   171
   example estimates   172
   factors to consider   170– 172
   manufacturer claim   171
   number of replicate measurements   172

purpose   168
quantity to be estimated   172
spiked sample   170
   definition   171
summary comments   173
time period of study   172
verification of manufacturer claims   173
zero standard   171
Dewitte   212, 216, 217
difference plot   74, 77, 79, 127, 132,
   150, 204, 213, 215, 217, 231, 238
diluent for use with patient specimens   106
discrepant results   128
dispersion   85
distribution   31- 32, 77, 86, 181
distribution statistics   74
duplicate measurements   160
duplicates of fresh patient samples   117

E

Ehrmeyer   37
enzyme methods   183
EP5   120, 223
EP6   106
EP9   223
EP15   120, 133, 222, 242, 263
   calculations using Excel   226
   precision data calculations   226
   precision protocol   224– 230
   purpose   222
   scope and definitions   223
   spreadsheet   226
   trueness data calculations   231
   trueness protocol using patient samples
      230– 231
   trueness protocols using reference
      materials   235
   verification of precision claim   228
EP17   168, 173
error assessment   28, 52, 188, 198
error detection   53
error framework   262, 264– 68
estimates of errors   214
evidence-based medicine   8
examination procedure   253
   ISO definition   256
expanded uncertainty 35, 261, 265

ISO definition   260
expected range   109
experimental data   11, 29, 62
experimental Plan   62
Expression of Uncertainty of Measurement
   252, 261
external proficiency testing materials   258
external QC   257
external quality assessment (EQA)   20, 58,
   189, 235, 257

F

F-table   94, 95
F-test   84, 89, 94, 94– 96, 96, 119
F-test interpretation   96
F-value   95, 119, 120
   critical   94, 95, 120
   observed   94
false rejection   53
familiarization period   66-67
   EP15   224
FDA   8, 42, 46, 67, 179
final method validation studies   66
final replication study   68
final studies   64
Fraser   23, 267-268
functional sensitivity   168, 170

G

Gaussian curve   86
general plan for validating performance   66
Goldschmidt Filter Model   9
good laboratory practice   168, 222
Guide to the expression of Uncertainty of
   Measurement   252
Guidelines for Verifying a Manufacturer's
   claims   222

H

Hagar the Horrible®   18
hemolysis   56, 68, 156, 163, 199
hierarchy of quality specifications   19, 265-
   266
high bilirubin   68, 163
high complexity tests   38, 154
histogram   74, 77, 118, 181

hsCRP   24
Hyltoft-Petersen   213, 218

I

immunoassays   183
imprecision   7, 16, 22, 31, 33, 63, 65,
    78, 94, 114, 115, 117, 119, 122,
    162, 192, 199, 203, 217, 254,
    256, 263, 266, 268
inaccuracy   7, 16, 22, 31, 32, 33, 63,
    124, 129, 131, 192, 199, 202, 263
    see also accuracy, bias
Inner, Hidden, Deeper, Secret Meaning   28
intended customers   262– 264
intended use   255-256
intercept   29, 81, 129, 182, 216
interference   34, 54, 56, 62, 66, 67,
    68, 201, 202, 253, 256, 266
interference study   43, 65-68, 87-88, 125,
    154, 166, 199, 201, 205, 256, 266
  comparative method   157
  concentration of interferer material   156
  criterion for acceptable performance   158
  data calculations   157
  inteferer solution   155
  interferences to be tested   156
  pipetting performance   156
  purpose   154
  replicates   155
  summary comments   162– 163
  volume of interferer addition   156
interferer solution   155
Interfering substances   48
internal QC   257
interpretation of test results   30
ISO   34, 252– 270
  guidance for method validation and quality
    control   252– 255
ISO 15189   34, 252, 252– 255, 262,
    264, 269
  calibration of systems   254-255
  validation and verification   253-254, 255-
    256

L

Laboratory Accreditation Program   47
laboratory processes   15
laboratory proficiency testing   244
laboratory services   17
least squares analysis, line   96, 129
Limit of Blank (LoB) 168, 170
  definition   169
Limit of Detection (LoD) 168, 170
  definition   169
Limit of Quantification (LoQ) 168, 170
  definition   169
line of best fit   107, 109, 128, 212
linear range   105
linear regression statistics   77, 84, 96,
    129, 130, 132, 146
linear-data plotter   74, 76
linearity   102, 112, 132, 148
  line of best fit   109
linearity study   42, 43, 102-105, 199, 205
            data analysis   107
            diluent   106
            materials   106
            number of levels   106
            number replicates   107
            procedure for dilutions   107
lipemia   68, 156, 163, 199
long-term imprecision   119
long-term replication study   126
Lucky Eddy   18
lyophilization   116

M

Making Sense of Statistics   147–150
manufacturer claims   46, 62, 120, 183,
    200, 224, 231, 242, 246
  for bias   233
  for precision   228, 230
manufacturer directions, instructions   41, 44,
    57, 224
manufacturer's method   200
manufacturer's reference range   198
matrix   115, 116, 125, 159, 201
matrix effects   78
maximum allowable bias   22, 249
maximum allowable CV   22, 249

mean   32, 77, 84, 85, 88, 90, 91,
    97, 107, 114, 118, 120, 122, 181,
    201, 202, 215, 217
        definition   85
measurand
    ISO definition   257
measurement uncertainty   35, 237, 259,
    252– 261, 263-264, 265, 269
medical decision concentration, medical
    decision level   68, 98, 117, 129,
    132, 149, 190, 201, 206, 215-217,
    246
medical usefulness   53, 76
medically allowable error   188
medically allowable standard deviations
    (SD)   19
medically important changes   21, 23
medically important decision levels   117,
    129
medically important errors   11, 21
method acceptability   68, 76, 78, 93,
    96, 131, 149, 150, 217
method characteristics   53-55, 199
method comparison data, study,
        see comparison of methods study
method decision   66
Method Decision Chart   75, 76, 119,
    132, 151, 190, 200, 202, 204, 242
  calculator 195
  example applications   193
  excellent performance   192
  good performance   192
  how to construct   190– 191
  how to use   192
  marginal performance   192
  poor performance   192
  unacceptable performance   192
  world class performance   192
method implementation   69
method performance   7, 11, 18, 33, 53,
    62, 64, 69, 79, 116, 150, 188,
    198, 200, 214
method selection   52–59, 214
method stability   102
method validation   28, 29, 34, 52, 62,
    69, 115, 218 11, 29, 30, 31
  applications with published data   200
methodology characteristics   54, 55, 56,

57, 62, 203, 214
minimum detection limit   168
moderate complexity tests   38, 67, 154
modern myths of quality   3-12
modified methods   199
multitest systems   57

N

narrow range of data   148
NCEP   117
Nevalainen   243, 244, 245
New York   38
non-linearity   148, 216
non-waived   34, 38, 40, 199
non-waived methods approved by FDA   41,
    42, 46, 47, 48, 67
non-waived methods not approved by FDA
    42, 48
non-waived tests modified or developed in-
        house   42
nonparametric statistics   86
normal curve   86
Normalized Operating Point Calculator   195
null hypothesis   89, 92, 94
number of measurements   119
numbers of control measurements   205

O

observed error   29, 76, 214
observed imprecision   79
observed inaccuracy   79
observed recovery   161
operating point   79, 131, 192, 203
operating protocol   66, 67
operating specifications   20, 21, 22
ordinary linear regression,
        see linear regression
outliers   78, 126, 132, 148, 216

P

paired data calculator   74, 77, 231
paired t-test   84, 90, 141, 215, 231
        calculations   231
        statistics   237
parametric statistics   86

Passing-Bablock regression   78, 149,
     151, 212
           technique   217
patient pools   105, 116, 117, 155
patient samples   124
patient specimens   118, 125, 127, 132,
     155-156, 160, 165, 166, 201, 202,
     218, 247
patient validation   10
Pearson product moment
     see correlation coefficient
performance   30, 34, 53, 54
performance characteristics   54, 55, 56,
     62, 203
performance specification requirements   48
periodic validation   45
pH   93
pipetting accuracy   159
pipetting performance   156
Plebani   9
point-of-care   54, 56, 212
points of care in using statistics in method
     valid   212–220
population of interest   84
post-analytic errors   8, 10
pre-analytic errors   8, 10
pre-analytical factors   22
precision   10, 33, 42, 46, 48, 54, 57,
     62, 66, 144, 156, 198, 222, 223,
     247, 263, 266, 268
   ISO definition   259
   see also imprecision
   see also random error
   see also coefficient of variation
preliminary method validation studies   66
preventive maintenance   45, 53, 69, 203
probability (p)   92
procedure, definition   39
proficiency testing   20, 45, 58, 189, 203
proficiency testing criteria   22, 23, 131,
     158, 189, 235
proficiency testing samples   133
proper use of statistics   219
proportional systematic error   31-32, 63,
     64, 65, 77, 128, 129, 139, 142-
     146, 159, 161, 162, 163, 199,
     202, 214, 215

Q

Q-Probe   244
QA, see quality assurance
QC, see quality control
QC procedures   18, 53, 66
QI, see quality improvement   16
QLP, see quality laboratory processes
QP, see quality planning
QS, see quality standard
quality   3, 6, 7, 15
   ISO definition   259
quality assessment   6, 16, 17, 39, 40
quality assurance   6, 16, 17, 18
quality control   7, 11, 16-18, 21, 22,
     43, 52-53, 69, 110, 224, 231
quality control materials   133
quality design   11
quality goals   20
quality improvement (QI)   16, 17
quality laboratory processes   16-18
quality management   8, 11, 15– 26, 219
quality planning (QP)   6, 16, 17, 18
quality requirement   7, 20, 21, 62, 163,
     188, 201, 246, 248
   analytical   188
quality standards   16, 17, 18, 21, 23
     a short history   18– 20
     convenient sources   23
     getting started   21– 22
     heirarchy   19
     trends and directions   24– 25
quality systems   38-39
quality-planning   18
     analytical   22
     clinical   22

R

random error   31-33, 63, 64, 65, 68,
     75-76, 91, 93, 94, 96, 107, 109,
     114, 115, 118, 122, 130, 132, 139,
     142, 145, 155, 188, 189, 190,
     198, 199, 203, 214, 217
     between methods   78
RE, see random error
reagents   56, 102, 201, 203
real world application of method validation
     198– 207

recommended tools for data analysis   73– 75
recovery   34, 54, 66, 67, 68, 162,
      163, 165, 201
recovery study   43, 65, 66, 67, 68, 87,
      88, 89, 125, 154, 158– 164, 160,
      199, 202, 205
      concentration of analyte needed   160
      concentration of standard solution   160
      data calculations   161
      factors to consider   159–161
      number of patient specimens tested   160
      number of replication measurements   160
      pipetting accuracy   159
      purpose   159
      summary comments   162–163
      verification of experimental technique   161
      volume of standard added   159
reference change value   268
reference interval   18, 42-43, 46, 47,
      48, 57, 66, 178, 182, 183, 198
      demographics   180
      establishment   179
      limits   181, 182
reference interval transference   178–185,
      179, 200
      approaches to consider   180–183
      background   178
      calculation from comparative method   182
      divine judgment   180
      estimation with 60 samples   181
      purpose   178
      verification by 20 samples   182
      verification with 20 samples   181
      what to do   183
reference interval verification   66
reference laboratories   258
reference materials   44, 133, 262
reference method   44, 124
reference range verification   42
regression analysis   99, 213
regression equation   96, 148, 183, 246
regression line   105, 143
regression line equation   97
regression statistics   74, 98, 147, 182,
      183, 190, 202, 206, 212, 215, 216
      application   98
relative values   107
repeatability   223, 227, 230
      definition   223

replicate measurements   31, 110, 155,
      160, 162, 201, 217, 228
replication   201
replication study   42, 43, 65, 67-68, 73,
      75, 95, 114, 116, 122, 131, 190,
      199, 201, 205, 246
      concentrations to be tested   117
      criteria for acceptable performance   119
      data calculations   118
      further considerations   120
      matrix of sample   116
      matrix of samples   115
      number of materials   117
      number of test samples   117
      recommended minimum studies   120
      time period   115
      total, between-day, day-to-day, within-day
         study   115
      verification of manufacturer's claim   119–
         120
      within-day   115
      within-run   115
      worksheet   204, 208
reportable range   42-44, 45, 46, 48, 54,
      57, 62, 66, 67, 68, 73, 76, 102,
      109, 132, 198, 199, 201
      definition   104
reportable range and calibration verification
      109– 110
reportable range study   102– 105, 199, 205
      see also linearity study
      plot 108
      worksheet 204, 207
residuals   29
Ricos   23
      see also biologic variation
      see also within-subject biologic variation
routine service, operation, or performance
      53, 66, 69
run   115

S

sample mix-ups   126
sample validation   9
SD, see also standard deviation   31, 33,
      93, 122, 188, 190, 192
SD calculator   74, 76
SD of the differences   78, 79

SE, see also systematic error   32, 33,
     129, 202, 215
selection of multi-test analytic systems   57
semi-annual assessment of accuracy   45
sensitivity   34, 168
sensitivity of statistics to types of errors   144
serum   116, 126, 160
short-term imprecision   119, 120
Sigma-metric   241, 244, 248
Sigma-scale   242, 267
simulation of errors in test results   138
single medical decision level   215
single vs duplicate measurements   125
Six Sigma   7, 79, 200, 242, 266-267
   A terribly short introduction   242– 243
   approaches for measuring process
        performance   243
   core principle   243
   example Sigma-metric calculation   247
   general guidance for calculation   248
   inspect outcomes   243
   power   248
   quality assessment of analytic processes
        246
   quality assessment of healthcare pro-
        cesses   249
   Sigma-metric calculation   246
   typical business performance   245
Six Sigma QC Design and Control   242
slope   29, 77, 81, 96-97, 129, 141,
     142, 182, 202, 216
smeas   see also imprecision, coefficient of
     variation, CV, precision   131
specimens   17, 31, 54, 56, 64, 65,
     66, 68, 116, 126, 154, 180-181,
     204, 218
spiked sample   200
spinal fluid   116
sresiduals   77
standard deivation for the intercept (sa):   98
standard deviation   29, 31, 75, 77, 84,
     85, 86, 87, 94, 97, 114, 118,
     119, 120, 129, 131, 145, 181,
     201, 217
standard deviation about the regression line
     97
standard deviation

definition   84, 85
standard deviation for the slope (sb)   98
standard deviation of residuals   97
standard deviation of the differences   90,
     93, 130, 141, 145, 150, 231, 233
standard error   97
standard error of the mean   84, 87, 91
   definition   87
standard laboratory process   16
standard materials   235
standard method validation process   15
standard methods   17
standard of quality   15
standard operating processes   17, 53
standard process for managing quality   16–
     17
standard reference materials   124
standard solutions   15, 116, 155
standard testing process   15
standard uncertainty   35, 237
   ISO definition   259-261
standards of quality   198
state of the art   22, 266
statistic, definition   84
statistical analysis   69
statistical QC   6, 8
statistical sense, sensitivity and significance
     138–152
statistically significant   79, 89, 92, 94,
     131, 141, 149
statistics   6, 28, 29, 30, 72-74, 84, 98,
     129, 183, 202, 212, 214, 219
Stockholm Consensus Conference   19, 265-
     266
Stockl   212, 216, 217
sy/x   78, 97, 129
systematic error (SE)   31, 32, 33, 63,
     66, 69, 74-75, 77, 87, 88, 89,
     91, 92, 93, 98, 107, 124, 125,
     129, 131, 132, 144, 148, 154,
     160, 188, 189, 190, 198, 199,
     202, 214, 215, 217
systematic shift   32

T

t-table   91, 92
t-test   89, 90, 92, 130, 143, 146, 215,
     217

analysis   144, 215
statistics   74, 77, 78, 138, 146,
    147, 149, 151, 163, 202, 206,
    216, 217
t-value   78, 79, 87, 90, 91, 92,
    93, 130, 142, 149, 150, 229
        critical   92
        observed   92
target measurement uncertainty 259-261
    ISO definition   259
target value   189
TE see total error
TEa see total allowable error   131, 190,
    191, 201
TEcalc   131
technical validation   9
test complexity   41
test interpretation   29
test method   124
test performance   33
test performance history   47
test results   15-16, 21, 23, 29-30, 69,
    114, 119, 179
tests of significance   89
Thienpont   212, 216, 217
thyroid stimulating hormone   189
tolerance limits   266
Tonks   18
total allowable error   33, 69, 173, 189,
    198, 214
total biologic goals   22
total error   19, 31, 33, 130, 131, 189,
    215, 262-267, 269
total laboratory variance   226
total quality management (TQM)   7, 17, 242
total replication study   66
total standard deviation   119
total testing process   8, 9, 38, 39
total variance   228
TQM see total quality management
traceability, traceable value   34, 256– 258,
    265
transference   179
translating performance claims into Sigma
    metrics   242
transposition errors   126
true mean   84, 88
true standard deviation   84

true value   258
trueness 34, 222, 224, 235, 256– 258,
    262, 263, 269
    EP15 definition   223
trueness of measurement
    ISO definition   257
turnaround time   15, 16, 17, 54, 56
type A uncertainty
    ISO definition   260
type B uncertainty
    ISO definition   260

U

uncertainty   34, 35, 237, 259-261
uncertainty of measurement 34
    ISO definition   259
unmodified non-waived methods   67
urine   116
user validation of trueness and precision   67

V

validation plan   203
validation process   53
validation studies   62, 201
    adaptations for individual laboratories
        205– 206
variance   94, 237, 261
variation   115, 118
verification of performance specifications   41
verification value   228, 230

W

waived tests   41, 46, 47
Walking tour of the validation plan   67
whole blood   116, 157
within-laboratory imprecision (CV)   226-228,
    230, 237
    EP15 definition   223
within-laboratory SD   226
within-run imprecision   65, 68, 229
within-run replication study   66
within-run variance   226-229
within-subject biologic variation   22, 271
working range   68, 103
world class quality, see also Six Sigma   242